Keto Air Fryer Cookbook

1200 Days of Quick, Tasty & Wholesome, Low-Carb Fried Recipes to Lose Weight, Boost Your Immune System, Improve Your Energy Levels & Heal Your Body From The Inside Out

By

Kendra Reeves

© Copyright 2023 by (_Kendra Reeves_) - All rights reserved.

This document is geared towards providing exact and reliable information in regard to the topic and issue covered. The publication is sold with the idea that the publisher is not required to render accounting, officially permitted, or otherwise, qualified services. If advice is necessary, legal, or professional, a practiced individual in the profession should be ordered.

- From a Declaration of Principles, which was accepted and approved equally by a Committee of the American Bar Association and a Committee of Publishers and Associations. In no way is it legal to reproduce, duplicate, or transmit any part of this document in either electronic means or in printed format. Recording of this publication is strictly prohibited, and any storage of this document is not allowed unless with written permission from the publisher. All rights reserved. The information provided herein is stated to be truthful and consistent, in that any liability, in terms of inattention or otherwise, by any usage or abuse of any policies, processes, or directions contained within is the solitary and utter responsibility of the recipient reader. Under no circumstances will any legal responsibility or blame be held against the publisher for any reparation, damages, or monetary loss due to the information herein, either directly or indirectly. Respective authors own all copyrights not held by the publisher. The information herein is offered for informational purposes solely and is universal as so. The presentation of the information is without contract or any type of guarantee assurance. The trademarks that are used are without any consent, and the publication of the trademark is without permission or backing by the trademark owner. All trademarks and brands within this book are for clarifying purposes only and are owned by the owners themselves, not affiliated with this document

Contents

Introduction 10
Chapter 1: Keto Explained 11
    1.1 Keto Basics 11
        1.1.1 Macronutrient Profile 11
        1.1.2 Is There Any Evidence That The Keto Diet Can Aid In Weight Loss? 11
        Is It Possible To Consume An Excessive Amount Of Protein? 11
    1.2 What Are the Mechanisms Behind The Ketogenic Diet? 12
    1.3 How To Tell If You Are In The Ketosis State Or Not 12
        1.3.1 The Ketosis State And How It Affects Your Sleep 13
        1.3.2 Bad Breath 13
        1.3.3 Reduced Capacity for Hunger 13
        1.3 .4 Increase In Thirst 13

Chapter 2: The Health Benefits of The Ketogenic Diet 14
    2.1 Lose Weight More Quickly and In A Healthy Way 14
    2.2 Slimmer Waistlines 14
    2.3 Raised Levels of The Beneficial Kind of Cholesterol. 14
    2.4 Puts A Stop To Your Hunger 14
    2.5 Decreased Signs And Symptoms Of Diabetes Type 2 14

Chapter 3: The Air Fryer 15
    3.1 How Does the Air Fryer Work? 15
    3.2 Advantages of Using an Air Fryer 16
    3.3 Parts of Air Fryer 16
        Air Fryer Basket: 16
        Coil: 16
        Fan: 16
        Exhaust System: 16
    3.4 How to operate the Air Fryer properly 16
    3.5 Factors That You Need to Be Aware of Before To Using The Air Fryer 17
        3.5.1 Helpful Hints for Cooking: 17
        3.5.3 Safeguard Tips: 17

3.5.3 Accessories for the Air Fryer: Hints and Suggestions 18

3.5.4 Keeping it Clean and Maintaining It: 18

Chapter 4: Breakfast 19

1. Crustless Quiche Lorraine 19
2. Avocado & Cheese Omelet..20
3. Lemon & Blueberry Muffins..20
4. Grilled Pesto Salmon with Asparagus 21
5. Bacon & Egg Casserole 21
6. Chorizo Breakfast Hash 22
7. Cinnamon & Egg Loaf 22
8. Cheese & Mushroom Egg Cups 23
9. Raspberry & Vanilla Pancakes 23
10. Sweet "Bread" Pudding 24
11. "Rice" Pudding 24
12. Scrambled Eggs with Salmon & Avocado 25
13. French Toast 25
14. Bacon & Egg Muffins 26
15. Blueberry & Hazelnut Granola..26
16. Hard-Boiled Eggs 27
17. Sausage Breakfast Sandwich..27
18. Mushroom & Spinach Frittata 28
19. Cauliflower Bake 28
20. Zucchini Fritters 29

Chapter 5: Lunch Recipes 30

1. Cucumber Avocado Salad with Bacon 30
2. Keto Tots..31
3. Loaded Bacon-Wrapped Keto Tots..31
4. Tomatoes Provençal..32
5. Crispy Brussels Sprouts 32
6. Baked Chicken Nuggets...33
7. Egg Salad with Lettuce 33
8. Sesame Chicken Avocado Salad 34
9. Beef and Pepper Kebabs 34
10. Bacon-Wrapped Hot Dogs 35

11. Japanese Chicken Mix 35
12. Stuffed Meatballs 35
13. Steaks and Cabbage 36
14. Succulent Lunch Turkey Breast 36
15. Creamy Chicken Stew 37
16. Cheddar-Stuffed Burgers with Zucchini 37
17. Bacon Pudding 38
18. Special Lunch Seafood Stew 38
19. Air Fried Thai Salad 39
20. Curried Chicken Soup 39
21. Chopped Kale Salad with Bacon Dressing 40
22. Kale Caesar Salad with Chicken 40
23. Spicy Shrimp and Sausage Soup 41
24. Slow-Cooker Beef Chili 41

Chapter 6: Dinner 42
1. Shrimp and Cauliflower 42
2. Stuffed Salmon 43
3. Mustard Salmon 43
4. Flavored Jamaican Salmon 44
5. Swordfish and Mango Salsa 44
6. Salmon and Orange Marmalade 45
7. Chili Salmon 45
8. Salmon and Lemon Relish 46
9. Salmon and Avocado Sauce 46
10. Crusted Salmon 47
11. Stuffed Calamari 47
12. Salmon and Chives Vinaigrette 48
13. Roasted Cod and Prosciutto 48
14. Halibut and Sun-Dried Tomatoes Mix 48
15. Beet, Tomato and Goat Cheese Mix 49
16. Broccoli Salad 49
17. Brussels sprouts and Tomatoes Mix 50
18. Brussels sprouts and B utter Sauce 50
19. Cheesy Brussels sprouts 50

20. Spicy Cabbage 51
21. Tasty Lamb Ribs 51
22. Oriental Air Fried Lamb 52
23. Short Ribs and Special Sauce 52
24. Short Ribs and Beer Sauce 53
25. Sesame-Crusted Tuna with Green Beans 53
26. Grilled Salmon and Zucchini with Mango Sauce 54
27. Parmesan-Crusted Halibut with Asparagus 54
28. Beef Stuffed Squash 55
29. Greek Beef Meatballs Salad 55
30. Beef Patties and Mushroom Sauce 56
31. Beef Casserole 56
32. Lamb and Spinach Mix 57
33. Lamb and Lemon Sauce 57
34. Lamb and Green Pesto 58
35. Burgundy Beef Mix 58

Chapter 7: Appetizers and Snacks 59
1. Mushrooms and Sour Cream 59
2. Eggplant Fries 60
3. Buffalo Cauliflower Snack 60
4. Banana Snack 60
5. Mexican Apple Snack 61
6. Shrimp Muffins 61
7. Zucchini Cakes 62
8. Cauliflower Cakes 62
9. Creamy Brussels sprouts 62
10. Cheddar Biscuits 63
11. Beef Jerky Snack 63
12. Honey Party Wings 64
13. Salmon Party Patties 64
14. Banana Chips 65
15. Spring Rolls 65
16. Crispy Radish Chips 66
17. Tortilla Chips 66

18. Zucchini Croquettes 66

19. Chickpeas Snack 67

20. Sausage Balls 67

21. Chicken Dip 68

22. Sweet Popcorn 68

23. Apple Chips 69

24. Bread Sticks 69

25. Crispy Shrimp 70

26. Coconut Chicken Curry with Cauliflower Rice 70

Chapter 8: Desserts **71**

1. Almond Butter Cookie Balls 71

2. Caramel Bread 72

3. Mini Cheesecake 72

4. Mini Chocolate Chip Pan Cookie 73

5. Pecan Brownies 73

6. Blackberry Crisp 74

7. Mug Cake 74

8. Pumpkin Cookie with Frosting 74

9. Cream Cheese Danish 75

10. Layered Peanut Butter Cheesecake Brownies 76

11. Toasted Coconut Flakes 76

12. Vanilla Pound Cake 77

13. Chocolate Cake 77

14. Chocolate-Covered Maple Bacon 78

15. Raspberry Danish Bites 78

16. Cinnamon Cream Puff 79

17. Pan Peanut Butter Cookies 79

18. Pumpkin Spice Pecans 80

19. Protein Powder Doughnut Holes 80

30 Days Meal Plan **81**

Day 1 81

Day 2 81

Day 3 81

Day 4 81

Day 5 81
Day 6 81
Day 7 81
Day 8 81
Day 9 81
Day 10 81
Day 11 81
Day 12 81
Day 13 81
Day 14 81
Day 15 81
Day 16 81
Day 17 81
Day 18 82
Day 19 82
Day 20 82
Day 21 82
Day 22 82
Day 23 82
Day 24 82
Day 25 82
Day 26 82
Day 27 82
Day 28 82
Day 29 82
Day 30 82
Conclusion **83**

Introduction

Although attempting a new diet might be exhilarating, it can also be stressful. There will be certain items you need to add, decrease, or modify from your current meals. Sometimes adopting a new diet may be as difficult as purchasing new ingredients and cleaning out your whole kitchen cupboard, or it can be as easy as purchasing only one or two items.

The ketogenic or "Keto" diet has gradually gained popularity over the last several years. It is a low-carb, moderate-protein diet with high-fat content. The body can easily transition from utilizing fat to utilizing carbs because of its almost ideal macronutrient ratio.

The human body depends heavily on fat and carbs to provide the energy it needs to function throughout the day. The Keto diet is intriguing because it may help the body to burn fat more quickly. Scientists have long observed that fat is the only factor in weight increase linked to several diseases, including diabetes, obesity, and epilepsy in children.

In addition to the ingredients, the manner you make your meals also matters. This procedure may be made a lot simpler by a variety of kitchen gadgets. Because of the miracles they can produce, air fryers are growing in popularity daily. With air fryers, you may prepare all of your favorite recipes in a completely healthy manner. Are you curious? A must-have kitchen device, an air fryer will guarantee that the hot air circulation within the chamber fries food. The hot air in the air fryer is circulated the meal at a high rate of speed by a mechanical fan. An air fryer only needs a few drops of oil instead of gallons. The biggest advantage of an air fryer is, without a doubt, that it uses less oil to cook, and because high-quality fat is so expensive, using less becomes one of the greatest reasons to use an air fryer rather than a deep fryer. Also, you may still receive the crisp texture of your meal that you might miss if you cut out carbohydrates from your diet. Yet refined carbohydrates are not required to make food crispy. Just an air fryer and this cookbook are required.

This cookbook will provide you with a 150-day meal plan for the keto diet and numerous meal options you may have yet to consider, regardless of whether you just purchased an air fryer or are an experienced air fryer chef. With a little imagination, everything is possible with this cookbook, from chicken to kebabs to sweets. Let us now demonstrate what an air fryer can accomplish for your keto diet. Enjoy the trip.

Chapter 1: Keto Explained

The ketogenic diet is predicated on the idea that the majority of one's daily caloric intake should come from fat. Because carbohydrates are the primary source of fuel for the body, eliminating them from your diet is necessary if you want your body to start using fat as a source of energy. But, in addition to those benefits, this regimen also has others.

Your liver will start producing ketone bodies as a result of following a ketogenic diet, which will cause your metabolism to shift away from utilizing glucose as the primary source of fuel and toward utilizing fat instead. — In order to attain this goal, the ketogenic diet keeps the consumption of carbohydrates below a particular limit, which is often set at 100 grams per day. Your overall health and how much weight you want to lose should determine the daily amount.

1.1 Keto Basics

The ketogenic diet has been used for a number of years, most commonly as a therapy for epilepsy. It is increasingly commonly used to enhance body composition, and there is some evidence that it may also help minimize the risk of some diseases associated with high carb consumption. On average, people acquire at least half of their daily calories from carbohydrates, while those following a ketogenic diet aim to consume only 5 to 10 percent of their daily calories for fuel. Because of this reduction, healthy fats can now be used as fuel in the body through the generation of ketones, which are molecules that are produced by your liver and turn fat into energy. Formerly, these fats would have been kept for an endless period of time.

1.1.1 Macronutrient Profile

On a ketogenic diet, the majority of your caloric intake will come from fat (75%), followed by protein (20%), and then carbohydrates (5%). (Each of the recipes in this book includes an indication of the amount of net carbohydrates and dietary fiber that it contains. Put these two figures together to get the total amount of carbohydrates. The amount of carbohydrate restriction necessary to enter ketosis, the metabolic state in which fat is converted into fuel, varies from person to person and is frequently dependent on factors such as insulin resistance, degree of physical activity, and previous experiences with dieting. If you are unsure about whether or not the ketogenic diet is good for you, you should discuss your individual nutrient requirements with your primary care physician, a nutritionist, or a dietitian.

1.1.2 Is There Any Evidence That The Keto Diet Can Aid In Weight Loss?

A common misunderstanding is that being in a state called ketosis is the same as being in a condition of weight reduction, which is frequently a side effect of following a ketogenic diet. The focus of your metabolism will most likely have shifted to fat storage by the time you reach the state of ketosis; however, you do not need to be in the state of ketosis or produce ketones for this to take place. Yet, following a ketogenic diet can assist in supporting a reduction in hunger and lower your demand for a continuous source of food. This is because the metabolic adjustments made inside the body when on a keto diet typically cause a decrease in body fat and enhance insulin sensitivity.

Because metabolic health, thermodynamic efficiency, macronutrient ratios, and micronutrient balances are all key aspects in weight reduction, you shouldn't place an excessive amount of emphasis on being in a state of ketosis if your primary objective is to lose weight. The most effective way to gain an understanding of how to make progress toward your goals is to consult with a nutritionist who has prior experience working with low-carb diets.

Is It Possible To Consume An Excessive Amount Of Protein?

The body uses amino acids not just as sources of nutrition but also as building blocks, and proteins are made up of a large number of these amino acids. These fundamental components are essential for maintaining good metabolic health, particularly when engaging in strenuous physical activity. The metabolic process known as gluconeogenesis, in which surplus amino acids are turned into glucose, can prohibit you from entering a state of ketosis known as ketosis deepening.

In order to determine your optimal level of protein consumption while adhering to a ketogenic diet, it is essential to consult with either your primary care physician or a nutritionist. Although your body might be able to satisfy its energy demands by burning protein so rather than fat, you shouldn't worry too much about protein influencing your degree of ketosis if you aren't following a strict keto diet.

The majority of the food on a typical Western plate consists of carbohydrates. When you ingest an excessive amount of carbohydrates, your body turns them into fat and stores the fat for later use as a source of energy. The goal of the ketogenic diet is to train your body to use fat for fuel rather than carbohydrates or protein. This is accomplished by restricting carbohydrate intake. Your body will simply utilize the body's own fat as fuel as necessary.

1.2 What Are the Mechanisms Behind The Ketogenic Diet?

Everyone is aware that in order to have energy, we require food. Your body will use glucose as its major source of energy if you consume a regular diet that is high in carbohydrates. It is simpler for your body to turn carbohydrates into glucose than it is to convert other types of fuel into energy.

Insulin will also be created in order to metabolize the glucose that is present in your circulation, and your body will retain the fats, which will eventually accumulate and cause a wide variety of health problems.

The ketogenic diet forces your body into a metabolic state known as ketosis, which forces it to make use of fats rather than glucose as its primary source of fuel. This is made possible by limiting your carbohydrate consumption, which, according to the theory, will result in your body being deprived of the glucose it requires.

Ketosis is a natural state that occurs in the body when the liver begins to metabolize accessible fats rather than glucose or carbs. As a result, ketones are created, which are then burnt by the body as the primary fuel source.

Your body will be forced into this metabolic function if you follow the ketogenic diet. This is the purpose of the diet. Because your body is built to adjust readily to a new metabolic state, the only thing you really need to focus on is sticking to the diet, and your body will take care of the rest on its own.

The ketogenic diet should not be confused with other types of low-carb diets. The distinction is that each day, between 70 and 75 percent of the calories in your diet should come from fat, 20 to 25 percent should come from protein, and 5 to 10 percent should come from carbohydrates.

If you follow these instructions, your diet will consist of a high-fat intake and a modest protein consumption, and you won't have to worry about counting calories because of this.

Because of how it impacts insulin and blood sugar levels in the body, protein consumption is restricted. When a person consumes a substantial amount of protein, the surplus of the protein is turned into glucose. As a direct consequence of this, your body will not enter a state known as ketosis.

Have you ever realized that if you have a yearning for food, you typically go for items that are high in carbohydrate content? This is because your brain has associated the starchy and sugary meals with feelings of ease and comfort.

The primary objective of the ketogenic diet is to consume an extremely low number of carbohydrates while simultaneously increasing the consumption of foods that are higher in fat and protein. In principle, if you reduce the amount of carbohydrates, you eat and enter a state of ketosis, excess weight should be quite simple to lose.

1.3 How To Tell If You Are In The Ketosis State Or Not

Regardless of whether or not you have performed any tests to determine whether or not you are in a state of ketosis, your body will exhibit physical indications to prompt you. It's possible that you'll have a loss of appetite, an increase in thirst, poor breath, and a heightened awareness of the scent of your urine. All of these are hints provided by your body.

1.3.1 The Ketosis State And How It Affects Your Sleep

If you have been in a state of fasting for eight hours or longer, then you are well on your way to burning ketones when you wake up after a restful night's sleep because your body is already in ketosis.

It will take some time until you reach the ideal fat-burning condition if you are new to the high-fat and low-carb diet. Your body has become reliant on the consumption of carbohydrates and glucose; therefore, it will not willingly give up carbohydrates and will instead begin to seek saturated fats.

Another common negative side effect is sleeplessness during the night. Vitamin supplements have the potential to sometimes rectify the issue that might be brought on by a decreased amount of insulin and serotonin. Try combining one-half of a tablespoon of fruit spread with a square of chocolate for a speedy solution.

1.3.2 Bad Breath

There is a possibility that you will taste something metallic or fruity, and the stench will remind you of nail paint remover. The fact that this is the by-product of acetoacetic acid, often known as acetone, is a very clear signal. You may also notice that your mouth feels drier than usual. As a natural byproduct of your body breaking down these high-fat foods, you can expect to see these changes.

The symptoms of foul breath will go away once you have been acclimated to the procedures included in the ketogenic diet.

When you are out with friends, opt for a diet Coke or a drink that does not include any sugar. In a pinch, you can also chew sugar-free gum. Constantly check the nutrition labels for the facts regarding the carbohydrate content; you might be surprised by what you find. Due to the fact that they cause ketones to be depleted, the Keto diet does not permit these. Because of this, you should only use it briefly. If you are currently at home, all you need to do is grab your toothbrush.

1.3.3 Reduced Capacity for Hunger

If you cut back on your consumption of carbohydrates and proteins, you will naturally consume more fat. The numerous fiber vegetables, lipids, and satiating elements that are offered in the new diet are the primary contributors to the decreased hunger.

Feeling "full" while adhering to the ketogenic diet is a significant advantage. You won't have to worry about being hungry, which is one burden lifted off your shoulders.

1.3 .4 Increase In Thirst

Consuming carbs causes an increase in the body's ability to hold onto fluid. The loss of water weight occurs after the carbohydrates have been washed away. As it is likely that you are dehydrated, you can restore some equilibrium by drinking additional water.

While you are putting away carbohydrates while on the ketogenic diet, you are encouraged to drink more water. If you are dehydrated, your body can use the carbohydrates it has stored to bring you back up to a normal level of hydration. When your body is in a state of ketosis, the carbs are eliminated, and it does not have the water reserves that it normally does. If you have tried prior diets, you may have experienced dehydration; but the greater carbohydrate counts prevented you from feeling thirsty while you were on those diets. As a result of this, the keto state is a diuretic state; therefore, it is important to drink a lot of water every day.

Chapter 2: The Health Benefits of The Ketogenic Diet

2.1 Lose Weight More Quickly and In A Healthy Way

Cutting out on carbohydrates is the most effective and sure-fire method for losing weight quickly. To begin, a diet low in carbohydrates, such as the ketogenic diet, helps your body get rid of any excess water that it may be holding. You will find that you have lost some water weight during the course of the treatment. In addition, because the Ketogenic diet decreases insulin levels, your kidneys will begin flushing out extra sodium, which will cause you to lose weight rapidly within the first two weeks of following the diet.

You will keep losing weight on the ketogenic diet for as long as you follow it religiously, right up until the point where you reach your target weight.

2.2 Slimmer Waistlines

You have different kinds of fat in different parts of your body. The specific areas of your body in which fat is accumulated are the factors that will influence how adversely your weight impacts your health. There is fat that is kept under the skin, known as subcutaneous fat, and there is fat that is stored within the abdominal cavity, known as visceral fat.

Because it has the propensity to collect around your organs, visceral fat poses a health risk. It is believed that fat around the abdomen is the primary cause of chronic diseases since it can feed insulin resistance and inflammation and is the principal cause of both of these conditions. As you start following the Ketogenic diet, you will notice that your waistline is getting smaller. This is due to the fact that the Ketogenic diet is particularly successful at lowering visceral fat.

2.3 Raised Levels of The Beneficial Kind of Cholesterol.

The term "good cholesterol" actually comes from the scientific term "high-density lipoprotein" (HDL).

The Ketogenic diet is associated with an increase in good cholesterol levels because it causes the body to carry the Low-Density Lipoprotein (LDL), also known as the "bad cholesterol," away from the body and into the liver, where it is recycled and excreted as waste. This causes good cholesterol levels to rise.

2.4 Puts A Stop To Your Hunger

The worst side effects of any diet are hunger and feelings of deprivation, which is one of the primary reasons why the majority of diets are unsuccessful. But, not the ketogenic diet. If you reduce the amount of carbohydrates, you eat and replace them with healthy fats and protein, it will take your body longer to digest the fats and proteins than it did the carbohydrates, and as a result, you will naturally consume less calories. In the end, you'll experience less hunger for a longer period of time and lose more weight!

2.5 Decreased Signs And Symptoms Of Diabetes Type 2

When you consume a lot of carbohydrates, your body will convert those carbohydrates into simple sugars.

As soon as this glucose enters your bloodstream, it causes an increase in your blood sugar levels and prompts the production of insulin in your body. As insulin is secreted, your cells receive the instruction to either take in glucose and utilise it immediately or store it as fat for later use.

Insulin resistance can be caused by eating carbohydrates of a poor quality on a consistent basis, such as white bread or beverages with added sugar. If this occurs, your cells will no longer be able to identify insulin, and it will be more difficult for your body to transport sugar from your blood into your cells. This is a contributing factor in the development of type 2 diabetes. To break out of this cycle, one must drastically reduce the amount of carbohydrates in their diet to the point that their body is no longer forced to secrete large amounts of insulin.

Chapter 3: The Air Fryer

You have made the proper decision if you are one of those people who enjoys the wonderful crisp of fried food and that "crunchy" goodness, yet, you steer away from those bad items.

It just takes a few minutes to prepare delicious and wholesome foods that have been air-fried thanks to the Air Fryer. We are certain that you will find using your Air Fryer to be a pleasant and simple experience. You are able to use your air fryer to make delicious and wholesome snacks that are a breeze to prepare because of the versatility of this kitchen appliance.

A device in the kitchen known as an air fryer, which cooks food by convectively circulating hot air around it while simultaneously applying heat to the food. The food that is cooked has a coating that is crispy on the outside as a result of the extremely hot air that is circulated around it, despite the fact that the interior is still wet and chewy. Because of its capacity to prepare extremely low-fat cuisine with very little or no oil while still preserving the authentic flavour of the dish, the Air Fryer has eclipsed all of the other cooking gadgets as the centre of attention in the kitchen.

Every one of the components of a dish is essential, but also the approach that is taken in its preparation holds a significant amount of weight. Because of its many useful features, the Air Fryer has become an essential cooking gadget for every modern home. You'll be able to prepare all of your go-to meals in a method that doesn't compromise on nutrition when you use an air fryer. It takes the role of deep frying and is a better alternative because it reduces the amount of fats used; the Air Fryer only requires a few drops of oil as opposed to needing gallons.

Through the use of a mechanism that circulates the hot air within the chamber, the Air Fryer successfully cooks food. Within the Air Fryer, there is a motorized fan that is responsible for recirculating the hot air at a high rate of speed around the meal. Also, you may cook, fry, roast, grill, and sauté with the Air Fryer all at the same time.

3.1 How Does the Air Fryer Work?

We realize that you are going to have a hard time wrapping your head around how the air fryer can fry meals without the need for oil. These cooking implements have names that are quite descriptive of their primary function, which is to circulate hot air around food in much the same manner that hot oil is used for cooking food completely through.

In addition to this, a chemical reaction that is known as the Maillard effect takes place as a consequence of this process. This effect takes place whenever an amino acid combines with a reducing sugar in the presence of heat. It causes variations in both the colour and the flavour of the meals that are consumed.

Due to the lesser amounts of fat and calories that are contained in air-fried foods, these are often touted as a more nutritious option to dishes that are deep-fried. This is a really good alternative to frying in oil at a high temperature.

To achieve a taste and texture that is comparable to that of dishes that have been deep-fried, air-frying only requires one tablespoon of oil as opposed to totally drowning the food in oil.

Advantages of Cooking with an Air Fryer People appreciate air-frying for a variety of reasons, but one of the primary reasons is that, in comparison to deep-frying, it results in a significant reduction in the overall number of calories consumed. Because you would be expending more calories than you took in, your fat-burning rate would increase proportionately to the number of calories you consumed. By utilizing an air fryer, the majority of people cut their calorie consumption by between 70 and 80 percent, on average.

In addition to this benefit, air fryers save a significant amount of time. Consider the fact that you can bake a chicken breast in an air fryer significantly more quickly than in your oven, and the resulting mess is often much simpler to clean up. During the baking process, this is a common benefit of using this device rather than a normal oven.

To reiterate, unlike deep-frying, air-frying only sometimes leaves your home smelling like fried food for several hours after the process is complete.

Another advantage of using the device is that if you live in a household with people who are selective about their vegetable consumption, particularly children, air-frying vegetables is a fantastic technique to give them a crispier texture and enhance their flavour.

The Greatest Foods for Cooking in an Air Fryer Potatoes and chicken are two examples of foods that, when prepared in an air fryer, tend to come out tasting even better than they do when fried in traditional oil.

We would suggest making sweet potato fries at home and air-frying them if you are looking for something to cook in the air fryer. With a traditional oven, getting them to the desired level of crispiness might be challenging. Instead, season them with your preferred rub, toss them in the air fryer, and savour the results!

3.2 Advantages of Using an Air Fryer

The following is a list of some of the advantages of using an air fryer:

- It is simple to clean.
- Healthy
- Saves time
- Simple to operate
- Saves space
- Many ways to prepare the food

3.3 Parts of Air Fryer

Are you a novice when it comes to utilizing an Air Fryer? To make appropriate use of it, you must first have a solid understanding of these components.

Air Fryer Basket:

The term "cooking chamber" may also be used to refer to this area. The sides are often made of coated metal, and the bottom is made of mesh. It is the location of the food preparation, and its appearance can change depending on the brand. A few of the brands have racks. These recipes may be used in any air fryer brand, so don't worry about whether or not yours is compatible.

Coil:

This component is also referred to as the heating element because it is responsible for producing heat thanks to the electricity that flows through it. After it achieves the desired temperature, the air is forced to pass through the coil in order to maintain it.

Fan:

The fan is essential for circulating the air and keeping it at an extremely high temperature in order to get your food to the desired crispiness. This is the component that is responsible for cooking the food.

Exhaust System:

The exhaust system eliminates potentially hazardous buildups of excess pressure, odorous gases, and filth so that they do not have an impact on the quality of your food.

3.4 How to operate the Air Fryer properly

If you are new to using an Air Fryer, it is quite vital that you handle the Air Fryer correctly, as this will make it much simpler for you to prepare the recipes. These suggestions are quite helpful.

Use Oils:

Keep in mind that you are on the Keto diet; therefore, the oil that you use must be suitable for usage on the keto diet. Olive oil, coconut oil, or another type of oil that isn't sticky can be used instead, depending on the recipe. Vegetable oil should be avoided.

Heat up the air fryer:

The majority of the time, prior to using the Air Fryer, it is necessary for you to warm the Air Fryer. It is imperative that you check out and adhere to the Recipes Procedures. If you make sure to warm the Air Fryer before using it, you won't have to worry about your food being overcooked because the Air Fryer will already be at the optimal temperature.

Prepare the Basket with Grease:

It is very crucial to grease the basket if you do not want the food to fall out of the basket. Even if you are coating the food with oil, the basket still has to be greased to ensure that the "breading" does not fall out of place. Always proceed in the same order as specified in the recipe.

Hold off on cleaning till later:

Wait until the Air Fryer has totally cooled down before attempting to clean it after you have turned it off. You will need to allow the Air Fryer a sufficient amount of time to cool down because it does not do so quickly. Before cleaning, you will need to set aside around half an hour.

Take note of the Cooking Time as well as the temperature:

Be sure to follow the instructions for each recipe to the letter. Each recipe calls for a different amount of time in the oven and a different temperature, both of which need to be adhered to precisely in order to ensure that the meal is cooked to the necessary level. It is possible that the recipe will require you to cook the food for a longer period of time in order to get the desired crispness.

3.5 Factors That You Need to Be Aware of Before To Using The Air Fryer

Before making your maiden voyage with the air fryer, you will need to...

1. Take off any and all of the package stuff.
2. Remove any labels or stickers that may be attached to the appliance.
3. Use some hot water, some dishwashing liquid, and a sponge that isn't abrasive to give the pan and the basket a thorough cleaning.
4. With a damp cloth, wipe down the interior as well as the exterior of the appliance.

It's possible that your brand-new Air Fryer will give out a scent similar to "hot plastic" during the first few times you use it. This is quite normal for brand-new Air Fryer models because the material is being heated for the very first time. After the first few times it's been used, you won't notice it anymore.

3.5.1 Helpful Hints for Cooking:

1. To get a crispy texture, you can achieve this by adding a tiny amount of oil to the pan (around three to four tablespoons). Never fill the AIR FRYER to its maximum capacity, since this will cause it to malfunction. While removing the pan from the appliance, proceed cautiously because the contents, including the oil, will be quite hot. This is to ensure that you do not hurt yourself. Take care when you're in the kitchen.

2. If you want to steam your food, add a little water to the pan (around three to four tablespoons). Never get the Air Fryer too full, since this will cause it to malfunction.

While removing the pan from the appliance, proceed with caution because the ingredients, as well as any steam or water that may still be present, will be very hot.

3. In general, a shorter amount of cooking time is required for items that are smaller in size than those that are larger in size.

4. The "Settings" chart located on the inside back cover of the container provides instructions for preparing frozen items such as french fries, chicken nuggets, and fish sticks.

5. Snacks that can be cooked in an oven can also be cooked in an air fryer if the temperatures are correct.

6. For baking a cake or quiche or frying foods that are fragile or full, place an oven-safe dish made of glass, silicone, or metal in the basket of the Air fryer.

7. The air fryer can also be used to reheat food by setting the temperature to 300 degrees Fahrenheit for up to ten minutes.

8. To achieve the best possible end result and to reduce the risk of the components being fried unevenly, give the smaller ingredients a shake halfway during the preparation period.

3.5.3 Safeguard Tips:

1. Before it can be safely handled or cleaned, the device needs to have approximately half an hour to cool down.

2. Do not place the equipment on or near volatile items, such as a tablecloth or a drape. This includes keeping it at least three feet away.

3. Do not position the device so that it is pressed up against a wall or another appliance. It is recommended to provide at least five inches of free space above the appliance, as well as five inches of free space on the back and sides.

4. Ensure that nothing is placed atop the appliance in any capacity.

5. The device should not be used for any purpose other than what is described in the user manual.

6. Ensure that the voltage that is displayed on the appliance is compatible with the voltage that is provided by the outlet.

7. If the appliance's plug, cord, or any other component has been damaged in any way, you should not use it.

8. If the main chord is broken in any way, under no circumstances should you allow an unauthorized person to replace or repair it.

9. Be sure that youngsters are unable to access the equipment as well as its cords. A cord should never be placed on a surface that is too hot.

10. Do not connect the appliance to a timer switch located outside the appliance.

3.5.3 Accessories for the Air Fryer: Hints and Suggestions

1. To prevent damage to your workspace, always set the warm Basket and/or Pan on the Silicone Trivet after removing them from the AIR FRYER. This will prevent the heat from damaging your surface.

2. Although the objects can be cleaned in a dishwasher, it is recommended that you wash them by hand.

3. A set of eight baking cups made of silicone.

3.5.4 Keeping it Clean and Maintaining It:

Cleaning Procedures for an Air Fryer After each use, you should make an effort to clean the equipment.

Before beginning the cleaning process, check to see that the device has completely cooled down.

Also, when cleaning the pan or the basket, you should not use any cooking tools made of metal or abrasive cleaning substances because doing so may cause the non-stick coating to become damaged. Using this blueprint will assist you in maintaining an appropriate level of air cleanliness.

1. Unplug the main plug from the power socket, then wait for the appliance to reach room temperature before turning it back on. The pan should then be removed so that the air and the fryer can cool down more quickly.

2. Dampen a cloth to wipe off the appliance's exterior.

3. Use a not abrasive sponge, some dishwashing solutions, and hot water to thoroughly clean the pan, floating rack, and basket.

4. If dirt has become ingrained on the basket or the base of the pan, fill the pan with hot water and a little dishwashing detergent. Place the basket into the pan, and then let the pan and the basket soak for roughly ten minutes.

5. Use a cleaning brush and hot water to remove any food remains from the interior of the air fryer, then let it dry completely.

Take note: This particular action on your part contributes to conserving natural resources. When the device has reached the end of its useful life, please do not dispose of it in the trash together with other common home waste; rather, take it to a designated collection location where it can be recycled.

Chapter 4: Breakfast

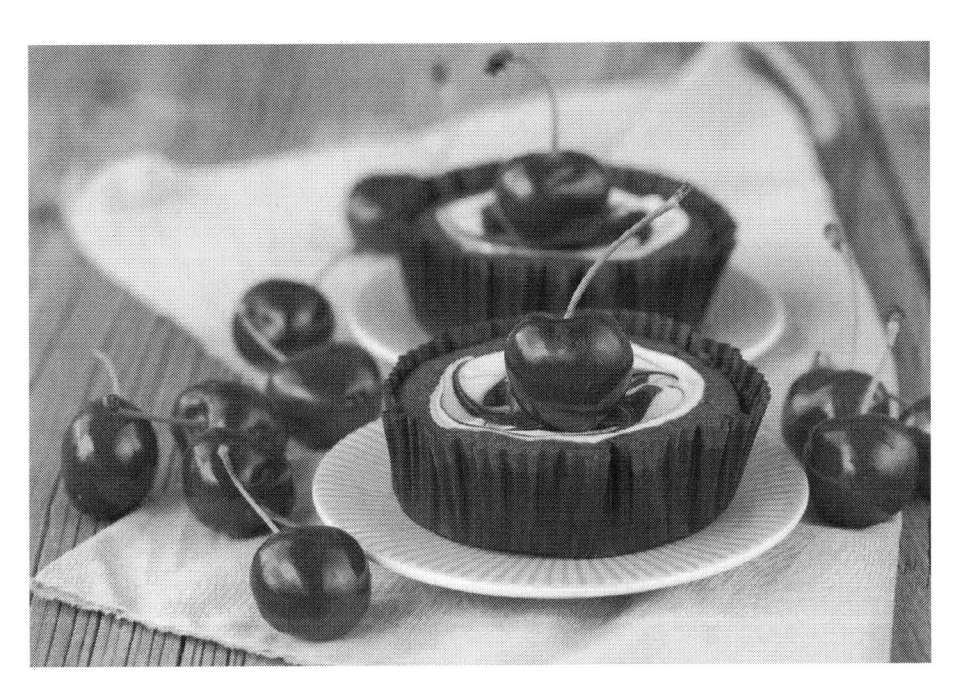

1. Crustless Quiche Lorraine

Preparation Time: 7 minutes
Cook Time: 17 minutes
Serving: 1

Ingredients

- 6 cuts of ham of 90 g
- 2 eggs
- ½ cup cream
- ¼ teaspoon paprika
- ¼ teaspoon ground nutmeg
- ½ teaspoon black pepper
- ½ cup and ¼ cup peeved Cheddar cheese

Instructions

350°F (175°C) should be the air fryer's temperature. Put the bacon in the frying basket and cook for a few minutes or until crispy. Place the cooled bacon on a platter. Smaller slices of bacon should be cut. Set aside. Place the ham slices in a circular pattern on the bottom of an 8-inch (20-cm) baking dish. Set aside. The eggs should be beaten together in a medium bowl. Add the pepper, nutmeg, paprika, and whipping cream. Blend thoroughly by whisking. On top of the ham, distribute a few pieces of bacon and the 12 cups of Cheddar cheese. Over the top, pour the egg mixture. Over the egg mixture, equally, distribute the remaining 1/4 cup of Cheddar cheese and finish with the leftover bacon. The dish should be wrapped in aluminum foil and placed in the fryer basket using the sling. Sauté for 12 minutes or until the quiche is well heated through. (Poke an egg to check if it is cooked and not runny. The dish should be removed from the fryer basket and let to cool for five minutes. Before serving, divide the quiche in half.

Nutritional Values:

Calories 573 , Carbohydrates 5g, Protein 31g, Fat 48g, Sugar 6g

2. Avocado & Cheese Omelet

Preparation Time: 5 minutes
Cook Time: 12 minutes
Serving: 1

Ingredients

- ½ teaspoon of oil
- 4 eggs
- 1 tablespoon of salted butter, liquefied
- ½ teaspoon salt
- ½ teaspoon black pepper
- ½ teaspoon basil
- ¼ cup of spinach
- ½ avocado 90g, carved
- ½ cup of peeved Cheddar cheese

Instructions

350°F (175°C) should be the air fryer's temperature. Apply the olive oil to a medium-sized pizza pan with a rim. The eggs and butter should be blended in a medium basin. Add the basil, salt, and pepper. Mix well. Fill the pan with the mixture. Top the omelet mixture with the spinach and avocado in an equal layer. Over the vegetables, smear the cheese. Place the pan in the fryer basket using an aluminum foil sling, and cook for 12 minutes until there is no longer any uncooked egg liquid or movement in the centre. (Poke an egg to check if it feels cooked and not runny.) After taking the pan out of the fryer basket, let the omelet cool for five minutes. Before serving, divide the omelet in half.

Nutritional Values:

Calories 421, Carbohydrates 3g, Protein 22g, Fat 35g, Sugar 6g

3. Lemon & Blueberry Muffins

Preparation Time: 10 minutes
Cook Time: 15 minutes
Serving: 7

Ingredients

- 1 cup of almond flour
- 1 teaspoon of baking powder
- 2 eggs
- 1 lemon
- 2 tablespoon lemon juice
- ¼ teaspoon of fluid stevia
- 1 teaspoon of vanilla extract
- 1 teaspoon of olive oil
- Blueberries (about ⅓ cup)

Instructions

The air fryer should be set to 320°F. The almond flour and baking powder should be combined in a medium bowl. Stir thoroughly to distribute the baking powder evenly. The eggs, lemon zest and juice, stevia, and vanilla essence should all be combined in a big basin. Mix well after adding the flour mixture. 7 silicone coats.

Nutritional Values:

Calories 157, Carbohydrates 5g, Protein 6g, Fat 14g, Sugar 7g

4. Grilled Pesto Salmon with Asparagus

Prep Time: 5 minutes
Cook Time: 15 minutes
Servings: 4

Ingredients:
- 4 boneless salmon fillets
- Salt and pepper
- asparagus, ends trimmed
- 2 tablespoons of oil
- ¼ cup basil

Instructions
Warm a grill to a high temperature and then oil the grates. Salt and pepper the fish, then coat it with cooking spray. The salmon should be grilled for four to five minutes per side until fully done. Oil the asparagus and grill until tender, approximately 10 minutes. Serve the pesto-topped fish with asparagus spears.

Nutritional Values
300 calories, 17.5g fat, 34.5g protein, 2.5g carbs, 1.5g fiber, 1g net carbs

5. Bacon & Egg Casserole

Preparation Time: 10 minutes
Cook Time: 30 minutes
Serving: 1

Ingredients
- 6 slices of bacon
- 1 cup of mushrooms
- ¼ onion
- ½ bell pepper, cubed
- 4 eggs
- 1 cup of cold cauliflower rice
- 1 cup of peeved Cheddar cheese

Instructions
The air fryer should be set to 400°F (200°C). In an 8- to 9-inch (20 to 23 cm) round baking dish with high sides, add the bacon, mushrooms, onion, and bell pepper. Cook the casserole in the fryer basket for 5 minutes, tossing halfway through, or until the bacon is crispy and the mushrooms are wilted. The dish should be taken out of the frying basket and put aside. 350°F (175°C) is the recommended air fryer temperature. Whisk the eggs in a medium bowl until fully mixed. Add the bacon, 12 cups of Cheddar cheese, cauliflower rice, mushrooms, onion, and pepper. Mix well. In the same baking dish, distribute the mixture, then top with the final 1/2 cup of Cheddar cheese. Cook the meal for 25 to 30 minutes after placing it in the fryer basket. Insert a skewer into the centre to determine whether the food is done. The casserole is prepared if the skewer emerges clean. The casserole should be removed from the frying basket and left to cool. Before serving, divide into four servings.

Nutritional Values:
Calories 320, Carbohydrates 4g, Protein 22g, Fat 23g, , Sugar 4g

6. Chorizo Breakfast Hash

Preparation Time: 5 minutes
Cook Time: 10 minutes
Serving: 1

Ingredients

- 1 bell pepper
- ½ yellow onion, diced
- 1 clove of garlic
- 1 tablespoon olive oil
- ½ tsp sea salt
- 1 tsp ground black pepper
- 5oz (140g) chorizo sausage, sliced
- 4 large eggs

Instructions

The air fryer should be set to 400°F (200°C). Combine bell pepper, onion, garlic, olive oil, salt, and pepper in a baking dish. To thoroughly coat the vegetables, continue mixing. Next, add the chorizo. Use aluminum foil to cover the dish. Cook the meal for 4 minutes in the fryer basket. Make 4 holes in the mixture after removing the dish from the fryer basket. Put one egg in each opening. In the fryer basket, place the dish once more, and cook for 5 minutes or until the eggs are cooked to your preference. The dish should be removed from the fryer basket and let to cool for five minutes. The hash should be split in half before serving.

Nutritional Values:
Calories 441, Carbohydrates 3g, Protein 23g, Fat 34g, Sugar 9g

7. Cinnamon & Egg Loaf

Preparation Time: 7 minutes
Cook Time: 35 minutes
Serving: 8

Ingredients

- 8-ounce cream cheese,
- 8 eggs
- 1 tablespoon jelly powder
- 2 tablespoon icy water
- 2 tablespoon warm water
- 1 teaspoon of cinnamon
- ¼ teaspoon of nutmeg
- ½ teaspoon of liquid stevia
- 1 tablespoon of olive oil

Instructions

350°F (175°C) should be the air fryer's temperature. Use a hand mixer to thoroughly blend the cream cheese and eggs in a large bowl, adding each egg one at a time until the mixture is completely lump-free. Set aside. Mix the cold water and gelatine powder in a small bowl. Give the mixture three minutes to rest. When the mixture is clear and fluid, add the hot water and stir. There ought to be no lumps remaining. To the egg mixture, add the gelatine mixture. Add the liquid stevia, cinnamon, and nutmeg. Mix well. Apply olive oil to an 8-inch (20-cm) square pan. Fill the pan with the mixture. Cook the pan in the fryer basket for about 35 minutes or until a skewer inserted in the centre comes out clean. After taking the pan out of the fryer basket, let the loaf cool for ten minutes. Slice before serving into 8 pieces.

Nutritional Values:
Calories 194, Carbohydrates 2g, Protein 8g, Fat 17g, Sugar 8g

8. Cheese & Mushroom Egg Cups

Preparation Time: 5 minutes
Cook Time: 16 minutes
Serving: 7

Ingredients

- 1 teaspoon olive oil
- 5 eggs
- ½ teaspoon paprika
- ¼ teaspoon salt
- ½ teaspoon black pepper
- 3 medium mushrooms, sliced
- ½ bell pepper, cubed
- ½ cup of peeved Cheddar cheese

Instructions

350°F (175°C) should be the air fryer's temperature. 7 muffin liners should be greased with olive oil. The simplest method for spreading the oil is to use your index finger. Whisk the eggs, paprika, salt, and pepper in a medium bowl. Put the same quantity of Cheddar cheese, bell pepper, and mushrooms in each liner. The egg mixture into each liner. Please make sure they are level and not pressed against the sides. Cook for 16 minutes, or until there is no movement or evidence of raw egg mixture when the sides are removed and the tops are deeper in colour. Before serving, remove the muffin liners from the fryer basket and let the egg cups cool for five minutes.

Nutritional Values:
Calories 80, Carbohydrates 1g, Protein 6g, Fat 6g, Sugar 4g

9. Raspberry & Vanilla Pancakes

Preparation Time: 5 minutes
Cook Time: 7 minutes
Serving: 8

Ingredients

- 8-ounce cream cheese
- ½ cup of coconut flour
- ¼ teaspoon liquid stevia
- 1 tablespoon of baking powder
- 1 teaspoon pure vanilla extract
- 4 eggs
- 1 teaspoon of olive oil
- 4-ounce raspberries
- 2 tablespoons of salted butter

Instructions

350°F (175°C) should be the air fryer's temperature. Blend the cream cheese, liquid stevia, coconut flour, eggs, baking soda, and vanilla extract in a blender. Once smooth, blend. Let the flour to absorb the liquid for five minutes by setting aside. Olive oil should be used to coat the sides of an 8.5-inch (22cm) round pan before adding the batter to produce two pancakes. Cook the pan in the fryer basket for around 5 minutes, or until bubbles develop and the sides are simple to lift using a spatula. After flipping, heat for another 2 minutes or more, or until well cooked. To make 8 pancakes altogether, repeat this procedure with the remaining batter. Put two pancakes on each of the four plates. 1 ounce (30g) of raspberries and 1/2 tablespoon of butter should be placed on each plate. Pour a little maple syrup on top (if using).

Nutritional Values:
Calories 400, Carbohydrates 9g, Protein 12g, Fat 33g, Sugar 5g

10. Sweet "Bread" Pudding

Preparation Time: 10 minutes
Cook Time: 22 minutes
Serving: 10

Ingredients

- 2 teaspoon of ground cinnamon
- 1 teaspoon of ground ginger
- ½ cup of erythritol
- 1 loaf of Almond Flour Bread
- 1 cup of whipping cream
- 1 cup of almond milk
- 6 eggs
- 1 teaspoon vanilla extract
- 2 tablespoons of cocoa nibs

Instructions

350°F (175°C) should be the air fryer's temperature. Blend the cream cheese, liquid stevia, coconut flour, eggs, baking soda, and vanilla extract in a blender. Once smooth, blend. Let the flour to absorb the liquid for five minutes by setting aside. Olive oil should be used to coat the sides of an 8.5-inch (22cm) round pan before adding the batter to produce two pancakes. Cook the pan in the fryer basket for around 5 minutes, or until bubbles develop and the sides are simple to lift using a spatula. After flipping, heat for another 2 minutes or more, or until well cooked. To make 8 pancakes altogether, repeat this procedure with the remaining batter. Put two pancakes on each of the four plates. 1 ounce (30g) of raspberries and 1/2 tablespoon of butter should be placed on each plate. Pour a little maple syrup on top (if using).

Nutritional Values:

Calories 300, Carbohydrates 5g, Protein 22g, Fat 22g, Sugar 7g

11. "Rice" Pudding

Preparation Time: 5 minutes
Cook Time: 10 minutes
Serving: 3

Ingredients

- 2 cups of rice of cauliflower
- 1 cup of coconut cream
- ¼ teaspoon of fluid stevia
- 1 teaspoon of cinnamon
- 2 teaspoons of vanilla extract
- ½ teaspoon of salt
- 1 yolk of egg

Instructions

Preheat the air fryer to 320°F (160°C) in temperature. Combine the cauliflower rice, coconut cream, liquid stevia, cinnamon, and vanilla essence in a sizable, high-sided baking dish. Mix until the colour is consistent. Put the dish in the fryer basket and cook for 10 minutes until the cream has thickened and the top has taken on a light brown hue. Take the dish from the fryer basket and thoroughly combine it with the egg yolk. Reposition the pan in the fryer basket, and cook for 2 minutes or until thick. Ensure the pudding is thoroughly combined before removing the dish from the fryer basket. Before serving, allow it to cool somewhat.

Nutritional Values:

Calories 440, Carbohydrates 9g, Protein 7g, Fat 41g, Sugar 2g

12. Scrambled Eggs with Salmon & Avocado

Preparation Time: 5 minutes
Cook Time: 6 minutes
Serving: 4

Ingredients
- 2-ounce butter
- 4 eggs
- 2 slices of cold-smoked cooked salmon
- 1 whole avocado, shared
- 5 chives, shared
- ½ teaspoon of sea salt
- ½ teaspoon of ground black pepper

Instructions
350°F (175°C) should be the air fryer's temperature. Put 30g (1 ounce) of butter in a baking dish with sides. To brown the butter, place the dish in the fryer basket for one minute. The eggs should be beaten together in a medium bowl. Cook the eggs in the dish in the air fryer for about 5 minutes, stirring once during that time, until they are soft and creamy. Take the meal out of the frying basket. Add the remaining 1 ounce (30g) of butter to the plate along with the salmon and avocado. To blend, stir. Before serving, top with the chives, salt, and pepper.

Nutritional Values:
Calories 480, Carbohydrates 3g, Protein 20g, Fat 43g, Sugar 3g

13. French Toast

Preparation Time: 5 minutes
Cook Time: 20 minutes
Serving: 4

Ingredients
- 2 eggs
- ¼ teaspoon of cinnamon
- ¼ cup of almond milk
- 10 drops of fluid stevia
- 1 teaspoon vanilla extract
- 4 slices of Cinnamon & Egg Loaf
- 1 tablespoon of powdered erythritol

Instructions
At 400°F (200°C), bake the food in the air fryer. Spray avocado oil on the fryer basket (or coconut oil). Whisk the eggs, cinnamon, almond milk, liquid stevia, and vanilla extract in a large bowl. Each cinnamon and egg loaf slice should be dipped in the egg mixture. 2 slices should be placed in the fryer basket in batches and cooked for 10 minutes, flipping once halfway through cooking. Before serving, place the French toast on a dish and sprinkle with the erythritol powder.

Nutritional Values:
Calories 584, Carbohydrates 9g, Protein 46g, Fat 41g, Sugar 3g

14. Bacon & Egg Muffins

Preparation Time: 5 minutes
Cook Time: 15 minutes
Serving: 6

Ingredients

- 6 slices of bacon
- 4 eggs
- 1 tablespoon of cream
- 2 tablespoons of water
- 1 teaspoon of ground black pepper
- 1 teaspoon of onion flakes
- ½ teaspoon of garlic powder

Instructions

The air fryer should be set to 400°F (200°C). Put the bacon in the fryer basket and cook for about 5 minutes, or until it is browned but still flexible. Take out the bacon from the basket of the fryer. Whisk the eggs, whipping cream, water, pepper, onion flakes, and garlic powder in a medium bowl. A slice of bacon should be placed inside each muffin tin before adding the egg mixture. Cook for about 10 minutes, or until a fork inserted into the side of an egg cup comes out clean. (Even though the top will appear to be cooked, the interior may occasionally require a little more time. Continue cooking in 1-minute intervals, testing for doneness after each one to see if the food is still raw. Before serving, remove the muffin liners and place them on a tray to cool for five minutes.

Nutritional Values:
Calories 95, Carbohydrates 1g, Protein 7g, Fat 7g, Sugar 8g

15. Blueberry & Hazelnut Granola

Preparation Time: 7 minutes
Cook Time: 7 minutes
Serving: 4

Ingredients

- ½ cup of almonds
- ¾ cup of walnuts
- ¼ cup of hazelnuts
- ⅓ cup of almond flour
- ⅓ cup desiccated coconut
- 1 tablespoon cocoa powder
- 1 egg
- ⅓ cup of salted butter
- ¼ teaspoon of fluid stevia
- ½ cup of blueberries
- 5 cups of almond milk

Instructions

The air fryer should be set to 400°F (200°C). In a food processor, combine all the ingredients minus the blueberries and almond milk. After roughly chopped and well blended, pulse. In a baking dish with high sides, pour the ingredients. Put the dish in the fryer basket, and cook for 7 minutes, or until aromatic and golden brown. Every 2 minutes, stir the granola with a wooden spoon to prevent the top from burning. The dish should be taken out of the fryer basket so that the granola can cool. 5 bowls should each contain the same amount of granola, followed by the same number of blueberries. Serve 1 cup of almond milk in each bowl.

Nutritional Values:
Calories 484, Carbohydrates 9g, Protein 14g, Fat 46g, Sugar 4g

16. Hard-Boiled Eggs

Preparation Time: 1 minutes
Cook Time: 16 minutes
Serving: 5

Ingredients

- 5 eggs

Instructions

Set 140°C as the air fryer's temperature. The eggs should be cooked whole in the fryer basket for 16 minutes. (Use a wire rack to lift the eggs out of the basket's bottom. Place the eggs in a sizable dish of ice-cold water. Before peeling, let the eggs cool for 3 to 5 minutes. Serve right away.

Nutritional Values:

Calories 77, Carbohydrates 1g, Protein 8g, Fat 5g, Sugar 9g

17. Sausage Breakfast Sandwich

Preparation Time: 5 minutes
Cook Time: 15 minutes
Serving: 2

Ingredients

- 9-ounce sausage
- 2 eggs
- ½ avocado, sliced
- 2 slices of Cheddar cheese
- 2 teaspoon mustard
- ½ teaspoon of sea salt
- ½ teaspoon of black pepper

Instructions

Preheat the air fryer to 350°F (175°C) of temperature. 2 egg rings should be sprayed with non-stick cooking oil. From the ground sausage into 4 sizable patties using clean hands. The patties should be cooked through after about 10 minutes in the fryer basket. Place the patties on a dish and leave them there. The egg rings should be put on a baking pan. In each ring, put one egg. Put the dish in the fryer basket and cook for 5 minutes until the eggs are cooked to your preference or have hard whites and slightly runny yolks. Each egg should be added to a sausage patty. One slice of cheese and half an avocado are placed on each egg. Each remaining patty should have 1 teaspoon of mustard spread on one side. Add equal amounts of salt and pepper to each patty. Each burger should be placed on top of a stack of eggs, avocado, and cheese. Serve immediately.

Nutritional Values:

Calories 680, Carbohydrates 8g, Protein 30g, Fat 55g, Sugar 11g

18. Mushroom & Spinach Frittata

Preparation Time: 5 minutes
Cook Time: 20 minutes
Serving: 1

Ingredients

- ¼ onion, diced
- 4-ounce mushrooms
- 2-ounce salted butter
- 2 cups of spinach
- 4 eggs
- 3 tablespoon almond milk
- 1 teaspoon of garlic powder
- 1 teaspoon of paprika
- 1 cup Cheddar cheese

Instructions

350°F (175°C) should be the air fryer's temperature. Combine the onion, mushrooms, butter, and spinach in a baking dish with high sides. Put the dish in the fryer basket and cook for 3 minutes, stirring halfway through, or until the onion is transparent and the mushrooms have slightly wilted. Mix the eggs, almond milk, paprika, garlic powder, and 1/2 cup Cheddar cheese in a medium bowl. Spread the vegetables evenly all around the dish after removing them from the frying basket. Over the top, add the egg and cheese mixture. Add the final 1/2 cup of Cheddar cheese on top. Put the dish back in the fryer basket and cook for 20 minutes, or until all the eggs are cooked through on the sides and in the centre. Before serving, take the dish out of the fryer basket and divide it into 4 halves.

Nutritional Values:

Calories 290, Carbohydrates 4g, Protein 15g, Fat 24g, Sugar 3g

19. Cauliflower Bake

Preparation Time: 7 minutes
Cook Time: 23 minutes
Serving: 6

Ingredients

- 2 slices of bacon
- 4 eggs
- 1 teaspoon of paprika
- 1 teaspoon of sea salt
- 1 teaspoon of ground black pepper
- 1 chicken stock cube
- ¼ cup of cream
- 2 cups of cauliflower rice
- 1 cup of Cheddar cheese
- 1 teaspoon of salted butter

Instructions

350°F (175°C) should be the air fryer's temperature. Put the bacon in the frying basket and cook for about 5 minutes or until crispy. From the air fryer, take out the bacon. Dice, then place aside. Whisk the eggs, paprika, salt, pepper, chicken stock cube, and whipping cream in a medium bowl. 12 cups of Cheddar cheese and cauliflower rice should be added. Mix well. Butter a high-sided 8.5-inch (22 cm) baking dish. Add the remaining 1/2 cup of Cheddar cheese to the cauliflower mixture before placing it in the pan. Cook the pan for 17 minutes in the fryer basket. Use a knife to pierce the dish's sides to check for doneness and ensure the dish's top layer is completely cooked. Make sure there is no undercooked egg mixture by poking the centre with a skewer. Before serving, take the pan out of the fryer basket and divide the bake into 6 halves.

Nutritional Values:

Calories 120, Carbohydrates 2g, Protein 7g, Fat 9g, Sugar 5g

20. Zucchini Fritters

Preparation Time: 35 minutes
Cook Time: 24 minutes
Serving: 14

Ingredients
- 6 zucchinis
- 2 teaspoons of salt
- 1½ cups of Parmesan cheese
- 2 eggs
- 1 teaspoon of ground black pepper
- 1 teaspoon of paprika
- 1 teaspoon of dried basil

Instructions
Grate the zucchini after trimming. Put inside a large colander. Over the top, evenly distribute the salt. Put aside for 30 minutes to allow the salt to suck out the water and the zucchini to soften. 350°F (175°C) should be the air fryer's temperature. By pressing the mixture into a colander set over a big basin or placing the zucchini in a clean cheesecloth and squeezing, you can try to extract as much water as possible from the zucchini much water as you can get rid of before beginning. Combine the zucchini, Parmesan, eggs, pepper, paprika, and basil in a big bowl. Mix the ingredients with your hands. Prepare 14 cakes of the same size. Place 7 or 8 patties in the fryer basket in batches and cook for 12 minutes or until well cooked. Before serving, place the patties on a tray and let them cool.

Nutritional Values:
Calories 108, Carbohydrates 4g, Protein 7g, Fat 6g, Sugar 5g

Chapter 5: Lunch Recipes

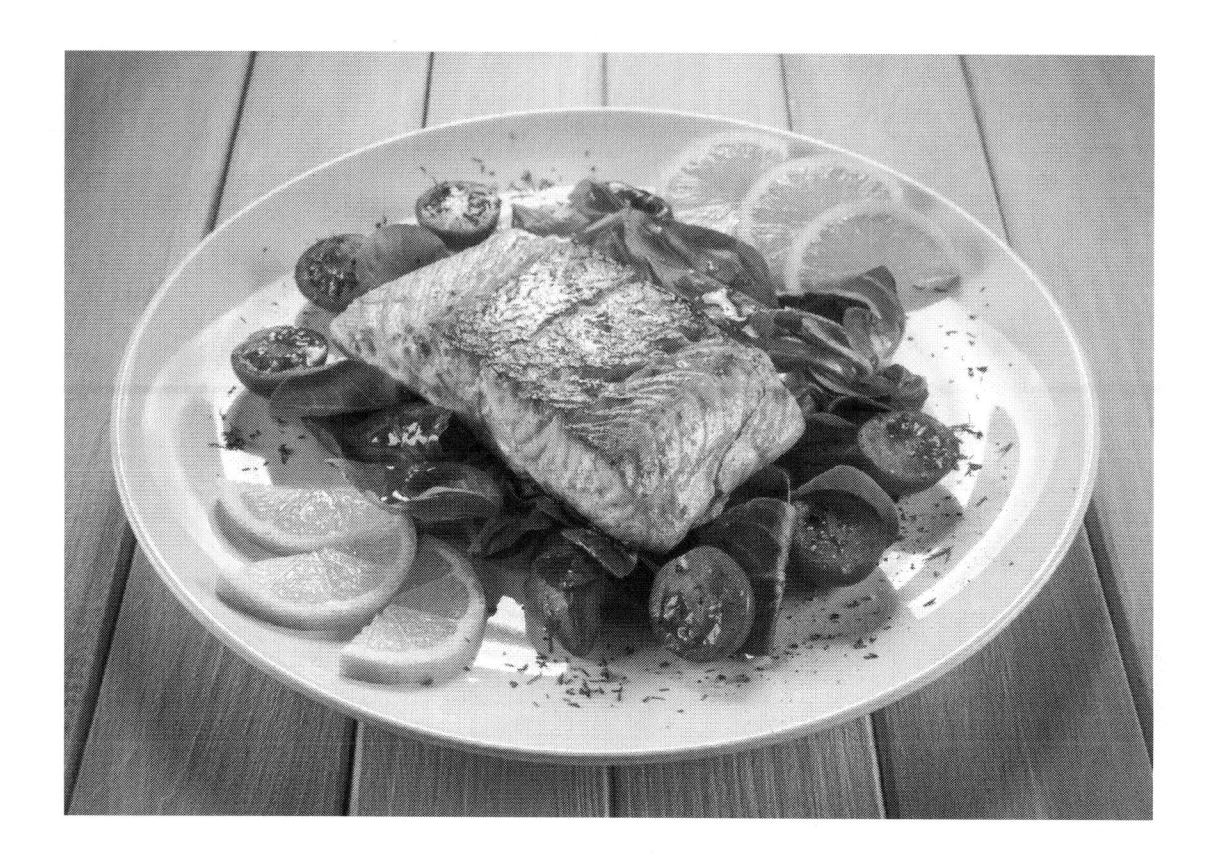

1. Cucumber Avocado Salad with Bacon

Preparation time: 10 minutes
Cooking time: None
Serving: 2

Ingredients

- 1 and ½ tablespoons of olive oil
- 2 cups of fresh baby spinach (chopped)
- ½ cucumber (sliced thin)
- 1 small avocado (pitted and chopped)
- 1 and ½ tablespoons of lemon juice
- Salt and pepper according to taste
- 2 slices cooked bacon (chopped)

Instructions

In a salad dish, mix the spinach, cucumber, and avocado. Mix it with olive oil, lemon juice, salt and pepper. To serve, add chopped bacon on top.

Nutritional Values

Calories: 365, Protein: 7.0g, Fat: 24.5g, Carbohydrates: 13.0g, Sugar 6g

2. Keto Tots

Preparation time: 10 minutes
Cooking time: 15 minutes
Serving: 6

Ingredients

- 3 cups of cauliflower florets
- 1 tablespoon of coconut flour
- 1 teaspoon of sea salt
- 1 egg
- 1 (8-ounce) cream cheese
- ½ cup of finely chopped onions
- 1 teaspoon of smoked paprika
- Chopped fresh parsley for garnish (optional)
- Ranch Dressing for serving (optional)

Instructions

Put avocado oil in the air fryer basket. Set the air fryer to 400°F for frying. The cauliflower should resemble rice grains after being processed in a food processor until that happens. Combine the riced cauliflower in a medium bowl with salt and coconut flour. Toss to coat evenly. Combine thoroughly before adding the egg, cream cheese, onions, and paprika. Cut 24 tater tot shapes from the cauliflower-cream cheese mixture. Leave room between them when you place them in the air fryer basket, and cook for 15 minutes or until golden brown.

The tots should be removed from the air fryer and put on a serving platter. If preferred, garnish with finely chopped fresh parsley and serve with ranch dressing on the side for dipping.

Remaining's may be frozen for up to a month or kept in the refrigerator for three days in an airtight container. Reheat for four minutes, or until well cooked, in an air fryer set to 400°F.

Nutritional Values

Calories: 166, Protein: 5g, Carbohydrates: 13.0g, Fat: 13g Sugar 4g

3. Loaded Bacon-Wrapped Keto Tots

Preparation time: 10 minutes
Cooking time: 13 minutes
Serving: 6

Ingredients

- 1 recipe Keto Tots
- 12 thin-cut slices bacon
- ½ cup of shredded cheddar cheese
- ¼ cup of sliced green onions (for garnish)
- ½ cup of full-fat sour cream (for serving)

Instructions

Put avocado oil in the air fryer basket. Set the air fryer to 400°F for frying. Each tot should have a slice of bacon wrapped around it, fastened with a toothpick. In the air fryer basket, arrange the wrapped tots with room between them. Cook the bacon for 10 to 13 minutes, depending on how crisp you want. After taking the tots from the air fryer and placing them on a serving tray, top them with cheese. Serve the sour cream with the green onions as a garnish.

When preparing these, remove the cheese from the cooked bacon-wrapped tots in an airtight container and keep it in the refrigerator for up to 4 days or the freezer for up to a month. Reheat for 5 minutes in an air fryer set to 400°F, or until crisp as desired, and then top with cheese as directed.

Nutritional Values

Calories: 385, Protein: 16g, Carbohydrates: 6g, Fat: 31 g Sugar 8g

4. Tomatoes Provençal

Preparation time: 10 minutes
Cooking time: 15 minutes
Serving: 4

Ingredients

- 4 small ripe tomatoes connected on the vine
- ¼ teaspoon of fine sea salt
- ¼ teaspoon of ground black pepper
- ½ cup of (powdered) Parmesan cheese (about 1 and half ounces)
- 2 tablespoons of chopped fresh parsley
- ¼ cup of Chopped onions
- 2 cloves of garlic
- ½ teaspoon of chopped fresh thyme leaves

For Garnish:

- Fresh parsley leaves
- Ground black pepper
- Sprig of fresh basil

Instructions

Put avocado oil in the air fryer basket. Set the air fryer to 350°F for frying. Without taking them from the vine, slice the tomatoes' tops off. Don't throw away the tops. To remove the tomatoes' seeds, use a big spoon. Salt and pepper should be added to the tomato inside.

Combine the cheese, parsley, onions, garlic, and thyme in a medium bowl. Mix well by stirring. Evenly distribute the mixture among the tomatoes. The tomatoes should be sprayed with avocado oil before being put in the air fryer basket.

Tomato tops should be placed in the air fryer basket next to the filled tomatoes, not on top of them. Cook for 15 minutes until the tomatoes are mushy but still maintain their form and the filling is golden.

Add a sprig of basil, fresh parsley, and freshly ground black pepper as garnish. With the tomato tops still on the vine, serve warm. Keep leftovers in the refrigerator in an airtight container for up to four days. Reheat for about 3 minutes, or until thoroughly heated, in an air fryer set to 350°F.

Nutritional Values

Calories: 68, Protein: 5g, Carbohydrates: 6g, Fat: 3g Sugar 11g

5. Crispy Brussels Sprouts

Preparation time: 5 minutes
Cooking time: 8 minutes
Serving: 4

Ingredients

- 2 cups of Brussels sprouts
- 3 tablespoons of ghee or coconut oil (melted)
- 1 teaspoon of fine sea salt or smoked salt
- Thinly sliced Parmesan cheese (for serving)
- Lemon slices, for serving (optional)
- Dash of lime or lemon juice

Instructions

Put avocado oil in the air fryer basket. Set the air fryer to 400°F for frying. Combine the Brussels sprouts, ghee, and salt in a large basin. Juice from the lime or lemon. After the Brussels sprouts are crisp, please place them in the air fryer basket and cook for 8 minutes, shaking the basket after 5 minutes. If preferred, garnish the dish with thinly sliced Parmesan and lemon slices. Fresh food is preferred. Keep leftovers in the refrigerator in an airtight container for up to five days. Reheat for three minutes, or until well cooked, in an air fryer set to 390°F.

Nutritional Values
Calories: 149, Protein: 14g, Carbohydrates: 10g, Fat: 12g Sugar 9g

6. Baked Chicken Nuggets
Preparation time: 10 minutes
Cooking time: 20 minutes
Serving: 4

Ingredients
- ¼ cup of almond flour
- 1 teaspoon of chili powder
- ½ teaspoon of paprika
- 2 pounds boneless chicken thighs (cut into 2-inch chunks)
- 2 large eggs
- Salt and pepper as per taste

Instructions
Set a baking sheet on the oven, preheated to 400 degrees. Combine the paprika, chilli powder, and almond flour in a small bowl. After adding salt and pepper, coat the chicken with the beaten eggs. After dredging the chicken pieces in the almond flour mixture, place them on the baking sheet. Bake until crisp and golden for 20 minutes. Serve warm.

Nutritional Values
Calories: 400, Protein: 43g, Carbohydrates: 1g, Fat: 26 g Sugar 10g

7. Egg Salad with Lettuce
Preparation time: 10 minutes
Cooking time: 0 minutes
Serving: 2

Ingredients
- 1 small stalk celery
- 3 hardboiled eggs
- 3 tablespoons of mayonnaise
- 1 tablespoon of chopped parsley
- 1 teaspoon of lemon juice
- Salt and pepper as per taste
- 4 cups of chopped lettuce

Instructions
The eggs have been peeled and cut into pieces. After stirring, add the celery, mayo, parsley, lemon juice, salt, and pepper. Spoon over freshly cut lettuce to serve.

Nutritional Values
Calories: 260, Protein: 10g, Carbohydrates: 3g, Fat: 23g Sugar 5g

8. Sesame Chicken Avocado Salad

Preparation time: 10 minutes
Cooking time: 0 minutes
Serving: 2

Ingredients

- 1 tablespoon oil (sesame)
- Salt and black pepper as per taste
- 4 cups of fresh spring greens
- 1 cup o avocado
- 2 tablespoons of oil
- 8 ounces boneless chicken thighs (chopped)
- 2 tablespoons of rice wine vinegar
- 1 tablespoon of sesame seeds

Instructions

In a pan over medium-high heat, toast the sesame oil. Add the chicken to the skillet after seasoning with salt and pepper. Sauté the chicken, often tossing, until it is well browned. After cooling a little, remove the chicken from the heat. Avocados should be placed on top of two salad plates of spring greens. Olive oil and rice wine vinegar should be drizzled over the salads. To serve, top with cooked chicken and top with sesame seeds.

Nutritional Values

Calories: 540, Protein: 23g, Carbohydrates: 2.5g, Fat: 47.5 g Sugar 12g

9. Beef and Pepper Kebabs

Preparation time: 30 minutes
Cooking time: 10 minutes
Serving: 2

Ingredients

- 2 teaspoons Dijon mustard
- 2 tablespoons olive oil
- 1 and half tablespoons balsamic vinegar
- Salt and pepper as per taste
- 8 ounces beef sirloin, cut into 2-inch pieces
- 1 small red pepper (cut into chunks)
- 1 small green pepper (cut into chunks)

Instructions

Combine the mustard, balsamic vinegar, and olive oil in a small bowl. Add salt and pepper to the meat before marinating it. After 30 minutes of marinating, thread onto skewers with the peppers. The Grill pan should be greased with cooking spray and heated to a high temperature. The meat should be cooked through after 2 to 3 minutes on each side of the kebabs.

Nutritional Values

Calories: 365, Protein: 35.5g, Carbohydrates: 5g, Fat: 21.5 g Sugar 3g

10. Bacon-Wrapped Hot Dogs

Preparation time: 10 minutes
Cooking time: 30 minutes
Serving: 2

Ingredients
- 4 all-beef hot dogs
- 2 slices cheddar cheese
- 4 slices uncooked bacon

Instructions
Cut the hotdogs in half lengthwise, through the thickness. Each hot dog should include a half-slice of cheese cut in half. The hotdogs are covered with bacon before being placed on a roasting pan coated with foil. Bake the bacon for 30 minutes or until it is crispy.

Nutritional Values
Calories: 500, Protein: 24g, Carbohydrates: 4g, Fat: 43 g Sugar 8g

11. Japanese Chicken Mix

Preparation time: 10 minutes
Cooking time: 8 minutes
Serving: 2

Ingredients
- 2 chicken thighs
- 2 ginger slices
- 1/8 cup water
- 3 garlic cloves
- ¼ cup soy sauce
- 1/8 cup's sake
- ½ teaspoon sesame oil
- 2 tablespoons sugar
- ¼ cup mirin
- 1 tablespoon of cornstarch
- Sesame seeds for serving

Instructions
Toss chicken thighs with ginger, soy sauce, garlic, mirin, sake, oil, water, sugar, and cornstarch in a mixing bowl, then move to a hot air fryer and cook for 8 minutes at 360 degrees F. For lunch, divide among plates, garnish with sesame seeds, and serve with a side salad.

Nutritional Values:
Calories 300, Fats 7g, Carbohydrates 17g, Proteins 10g, Sugar 5g

12. Stuffed Meatballs

Preparation time: 10 minutes
Cooking time: 8 minutes
Serving: 4

Ingredients
- 1/3 cup bread crumbs
- 1 egg
- 3 tablespoons milk
- 1 tablespoon ketchup
- ½ teaspoon marjoram
- 1-pound lean beef
- 20 cheddar cheese cubes
- 1 tablespoon olive oil
- Salt and black pepper to the taste

Instructions
Whisk together bread crumbs, milk, marjoram, ketchup, salt, pepper, and egg in a mixing dish. Add the beef, stir, and form 20 meatballs from the mixture. Each meatball should be shaped around a cheese cube then rubbed with oil. Place all meatballs in a preheated air fryer and cook for 10 minutes at 390 degrees F. Serve with a side salad for lunch.

Nutritional Values:
Calories 200, Fats 5g, Carbohydrates 12g, Proteins 5g, Sugar 8g

13. Steaks and Cabbage
Preparation time: 10 minutes
Cooking time: 10 minutes
Serving: 4

Ingredients
- ½ pound sirloin steak
- 2 cups green cabbage
- 1 tablespoon peanut oil
- 1 yellow bell pepper
- 2 green onions
- 2 teaspoons cornstarch
- 2 garlic cloves
- Salt and black pepper to the taste

Instructions
Toss cabbage with salt, pepper, and peanut oil in a bowl, then add to an air fryer basket and cook it for 4 minutes at 370 degrees F. Toss steak strips with green onions, bell pepper, garlic, salt, and pepper in your air fryer and cook for 5 minutes. Toss in the cabbage, divide amongst plates and serve for lunch.

Nutritional Values:
Calories 282, Fats 6g, Carbohydrates 14g, Proteins 6g, Sugar 0g

14. Succulent Lunch Turkey Breast
Preparation time: 10 minutes
Cooking time: 47 minutes
Serving: 4

Ingredients
- 1 big turkey breast
- 2 tablespoons mustard
- ½ teaspoon smoked paprika
- 1 teaspoon thyme
- 2 teaspoons olive oil
- ½ teaspoon sage
- Salt and black pepper to the taste
- ¼ cup maple syrup
- 1 tablespoon butter

Instructions
Dust the turkey breast with olive oil, and season with salt, thyme, pepper, paprika, and sage, rub and put in the basket of your air fryer to cook for 25 minutes at 350 degrees F. Cook for another 10 minutes after flipping the turkey, then cook for another 10 minutes. Meanwhile, melt the butter in a put over medium heat, add the mustard and maple syrup, swirl well, and simmer for a few minutes before turning off the heat. Slice the turkey breast, split among plates, and sprinkle with maple glaze.

Nutritional Values:
Calories 280, Fats 2g, Carbohydrates 16g, Proteins 14g, Sugar 3g

15. Creamy Chicken Stew

Preparation time: 10 minutes
Cooking time: 25 minutes
Serving: 4

Ingredients
- 1 + ½ cups canned cream of celery soup
- 6 chicken tenders
- 2 potatoes
- 1 thyme spring
- 1 tablespoon milk
- 1 bay leaf
- 1 egg yolk
- ½ cup heavy cream
- Salt and black pepper to the taste

Instructions
Toss chicken with cream of celery, heavy cream, potatoes, bay leaf, thyme, salt, and pepper in a mixing bowl, then pour into your air fryer's pan and cook for 25 minutes at 320 degrees F. Allow for some cooling time before discarding the bay leaf, dividing the stew among plates, and serving straight away.

Nutritional Values:
Calories 300, Fats 11g, Carbohydrates 23g, Proteins 14g, Sugar 8g

16. Cheddar-Stuffed Burgers with Zucchini

Prep Time: 10 minutes
Cook Time: 15 minutes
Servings: 4

Ingredients
- 1 pound of beef
- 2 eggs
- ¼ cup of almond flour
- 1 cup of cheese
- Salt and pepper
- 2 tablespoons of oil
- 1 large zucchini

Instructions
In a bowl, mix the ground beef with the egg, almond flour, cheese, salt, and pepper. Thoroughly combine, then form into four uniform burgers. Oil should be heated in a big pan over medium heat. Put the burger patties in and brown them for about 5 minutes. After you've flipped the patties, add the zucchini and toss to coat with oil. Add salt and pepper to taste, then boil the zucchini for 5 minutes, stirring periodically. Put the zucchini on the side and top the burgers with whatever you choose.

Nutritional Values
470 calories, 29.5g fat, 47g protein, 4.5g carbs, 1.5g fiber, 3g net carbs

17. Bacon Pudding

Preparation time: 10 minutes
Cooking time: 25 minutes
Serving: 2

Ingredients
- 4 bacon strips
- 1 tablespoon butter
- 1 + ½ cups milk
- 2 cups corn
- 1 yellow onion
- ½ cup heavy cream
- ¼ cup celery
- ½ cup red bell pepper
- 3 eggs
- 1 teaspoon thyme
- 2 teaspoons garlic
- 3 cups bread
- 4 tablespoons parmesan
- Cooking spray
- Salt and black pepper to the taste

Instructions
Coat the pan of your air fryer with cooking spray. Toss bacon with butter, corn, onion, bell pepper, thyme, celery, garlic, salt, eggs, pepper, milk, heavy cream, and bread cubes in a mixing bowl, then pour into a prepared baking pan top with cheese. Cook for 30 minutes at 320 degrees in an air fryer preheated. For a fast lunch, divide the mixture among plates and serve warm.

Nutritional Values:
Calories 276, Fats 10g, Carbohydrates 20g, Proteins 10g, Sugar 9g

18. Special Lunch Seafood Stew

Preparation time: 10 minutes
Cooking time: 20 minutes
Serving: 4

Ingredients
- 5 ounces white rice
- 2 ounces peas
- 1 red bell pepper
- 4 shrimp
- 14 ounces white wine
- 3 ounces water
- 6 scallops
- 2 ounces squid pieces
- 7 ounces mussels
- 1 tablespoon olive oil
- 3 ounces sea bass fillet
- 3.5 ounces clams
- 4 crayfish
- Salt and black pepper to the taste

Instructions
Combine sea bass, shrimp, mussels, scallops, crayfish, clams, and squid in the pan of your air fryer. Toss in the oil, salt, and pepper to coat. Stir together the peas, salt, pepper, bell pepper, and rice in a mixing bowl. Add this to the seafood, along with the wine and water, and simmer for 20 minutes at 400 degrees F, stirring halfway through. Serve for lunch by dividing the mixture into bowls.

Nutritional Values:
Calories 300, Fats 12g, Carbohydrates 23g, Proteins 25g, Sugar 4g

19. Air Fried Thai Salad

Preparation time: 10 minutes
Cooking time: 5 minutes
Serving: 4

Ingredients
- 1 cup red cabbage
- 1 cup carrots
- Handful cilantro
- Juice from 1 lime
- 1 small cucumber
- 2 teaspoons red curry paste
- 12 big shrimp
- A pinch of salt and black pepper

Instructions
Combine cabbage, carrots, cucumber, and shrimp in a pan that fits your air fryer, stir and cook at 360 F for 5 minutes. Toss in the salt, pepper, lime juice, cilantro, and red curry paste, then divide into plates and serve immediately.

Nutritional Values:
Calories 172, Fats 5g, Carbohydrates 8g, Proteins 5g, Sugar 11g

20. Curried Chicken Soup

Preparation time: 10 minutes
Cooking time: 20 minutes
Serving: 4

Ingredients
- 2 teaspoons of curry powder
- 2 tablespoons olive oil (divided)
- 4 boneless chicken thighs (about 12 ounces)
- 1 small yellow onion (chopped)
- 2 teaspoons of crushed cumin
- Pinch cayenne
- 4 cups of chopped cauliflower
- 4 cups of chicken broth
- 1 cup of water
- 2 cloves of minced garlic
- ½ cup of canned coconut milk
- 2 cups of chopped kale
- Fresh chopped cilantro

Instructions
Put the chicken aside after chopping it into bite-sized pieces. In a saucepan, warm 1 tablespoon of oil over medium heat. After cooking the onions for 4 minutes, toss half the spices. Cauliflower is added, and the cooking time is increased by 4 minutes. Add the broth, followed by the water and garlic, and bring to a boil. After lowering the heat, simmer the cauliflower for ten minutes or until tender. Remove from the heat and toss in the greens and coconut milk. Heat the remaining oil in a skillet and add the chicken; cook them until brown. Add the other spices and cook the chicken for a further few minutes. After stirring the chicken, serve the soup hot with fresh cilantro as a garnish.

Nutritional Values
Calories: 500, Protein: 24g, Carbohydrates: 4g, Fat: 43 g, Sugar 2g

21. Chopped Kale Salad with Bacon Dressing

Preparation time: 15 minutes
Cooking time: 0 minutes
Serving: 2

Ingredients
- 2 tablespoons of apple cider vinegar
- 6 slices of uncooked bacon
- 1 teaspoon of Dijon mustard
- Liquid stevia (up to taste)
- Salt and pepper
- 4 cups of fresh chopped kale
- ¼ cup of thinly sliced red onion

Instructions
The bacon should be cooked in a pan until crisp before being removed and chopped. 14 cups of the bacon grease should be saved and warmed in the pan over low heat. Add salt and pepper after whisking in the stevia, mustard, and apple cider vinegar. Kale should be added and cooked for one minute before being divided between two dishes. To serve, sprinkle chopped bacon and red onion on the salads.

Nutritional Values
Calories: 230, Protein: 15g, Carbohydrates: 13.5g, Fat:12g, Sugar 12g

22. Kale Caesar Salad with Chicken

Preparation time: 10 minutes
Cooking time: 10 minutes
Serving: 2

Ingredients
- 1 tablespoon of olive oil
- 6 ounces chicken thigh
- Salt and black pepper
- 3 tablespoons mayonnaise
- 1 tablespoon lemon juice
- 1 anchovy
- 1 teaspoon Dijon mustard
- 1 clove garlic
- 4 cups fresh kale

Instructions
In a skillet set over medium-high heat, warm the oil. Add the chicken to the skillet after seasoning with salt and pepper. Remove the chicken from the fire after cooking until the color is gone. Combine the mayonnaise, lemon juice, mustard, garlic, and anchovies in a blender. Add salt and pepper after blending until smooth. To serve, split the kale in half and add the chicken on top after tossing it with the dressing.

Nutritional Values
Calories: 390, Protein: 19g, Carbohydrates: 12.5g, Fat:30 g, Sugar 22g

23. Spicy Shrimp and Sausage Soup

Preparation time: 15 minutes
Cooking time: 30 minutes
Serving: 4

Ingredients

- 1 small yellow onion (chopped)
- 1 tablespoon olive oil
- 3 small stalks celery
- 1 small red pepper (chopped)
- 3 cloves garlic (minced)
- 1 tablespoon of tomato paste
- 2 teaspoons of smoked paprika
- ½ teaspoon of ground coriander
- Salt and pepper
- 8 ounces chorizo sausage (diced)
- 1 cup diced tomatoes
- 4 cups chicken broth
- 12 ounces shrimp
- Fresh chopped cilantro

Instructions

In a large stockpot, heat the oil over medium-high heat. For 6 to 8 minutes, until the vegetables are soft, add the celery, onion, and red pepper. After adding the spices, tomato paste, and garlic, cook for one minute. Cook the tomatoes and sausage for 5 minutes more. Add the broth, stir, and cook for 20 minutes, uncovered, at a simmer. Add the shrimp after adjusting the spice to taste. Simmer for 3 to 4 minutes or until the food is almost done. Pour into bowls, garnish with fresh cilantro, and enjoy.

Nutritional Values Calories: 465, Protein: 11.5g, Carbohydrates: 11.5g, Fat:39g, Sugar 8g

24. Slow-Cooker Beef Chili

Preparation time: 10 minutes
Cooking time: 6 hours
Serving: 4

Ingredients

- 1 tablespoon coconut oil
- 1 medium yellow onion (chopped)
- 3 cloves garlic (minced)
- 1 pound ground beef (80% lean)
- 1 small red pepper (chopped)
- 1 small green pepper (chopped)
- 1 cup of (diced) tomatoes
- 1 cup of (low-carb) tomato sauce
- 1 tablespoon of chili powder
- 2 teaspoons of dried oregano
- 1 and half teaspoons of dried basil
- Salt and pepper
- ¾ cup of (shredded) cheddar cheese
- ½ cup of diced red onion

Instructions

In a skillet set over medium-high heat, warm the oil. After adding the onions and cooking them for 4 minutes, add the garlic and cook it for 1 minute. Add the meat, stir, and heat until it is browned. Remove some of the fat before serving. Place the spices in a slow cooker after spooning the mixture in. For 5 to 6 hours, simmer on low heat with a cover before spooning into bowls. Serve with minced red onion and grated cheddar.

Nutritional Values

Calories: 395, Protein: 12.5g, Carbohydrates: 12.5g, Fat: 19.5g, Sugar 2g

Chapter 6: Dinner

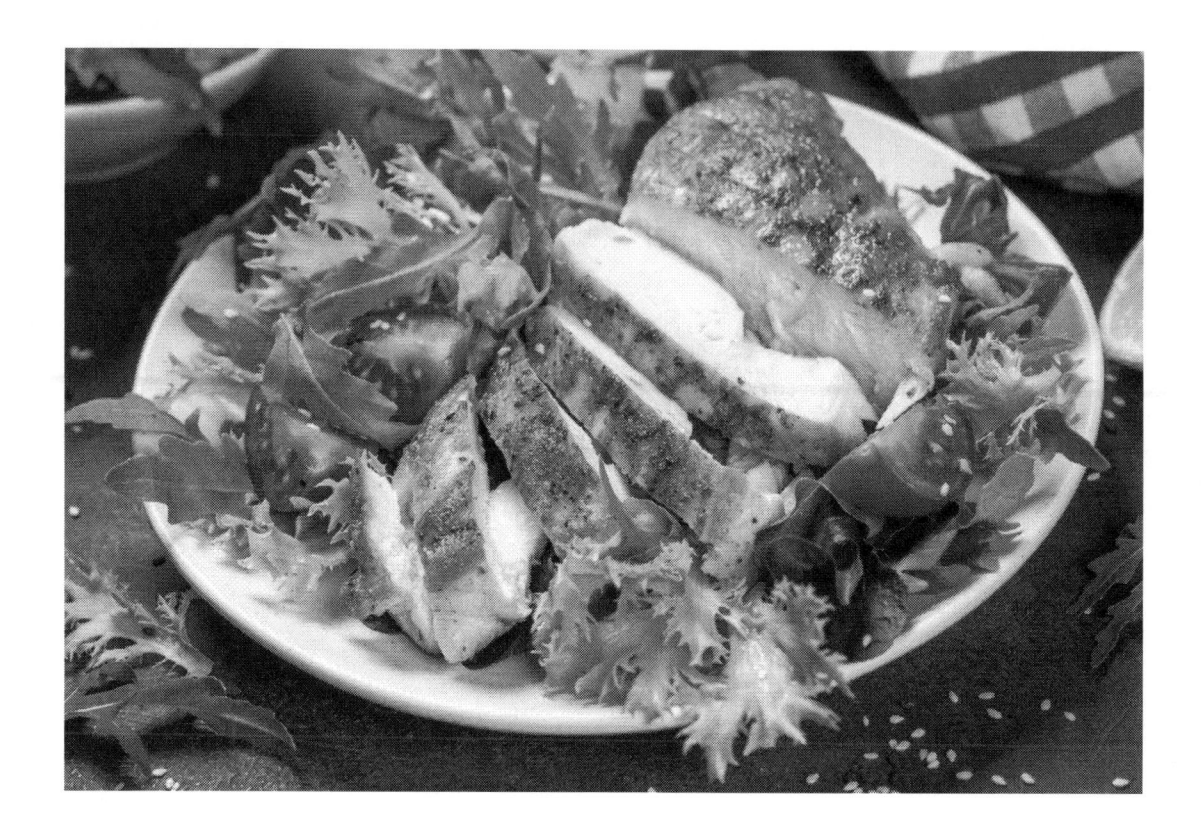

1. Shrimp and Cauliflower

Preparation time: 10 minutes
Cooking time: 12 minutes
Servings: 2

Ingredients:
- 1 tablespoon of butter
- Cooking spray
- 1 cauliflower head
- 1 pound shrimp
- ¼ cup of heavy cream
- 8 ounces mushrooms
- A pinch of red pepper flakes
- Salt and black pepper to taste
- 2 garlic cloves
- 4 cooked and crumbled bacon slices
- Half cup of beef stock
- 1 tablespoon of parsley
- 1 tablespoon of chives

Instructions:
Season shrimp with salt and pepper, spray with cooking oil, place in your air fryer and cook at 360 degrees F for 7 minutes. Meanwhile, heat up a pan with the butter over medium heat, add mushrooms, stir and cook for 3-4 minutes. Add garlic, cauliflower rice, pepper flakes, stock, cream, chives, parsley, salt and pepper, stir, cook for a few minutes and take off heat. Divide shrimp on plates, add cauliflower mix on the side, sprinkle bacon on top and serve.

Nutritional Values:
Calories 211, Fats 14g, Carbohydrates 8g, Proteins 3g, Sugar 2g

2. Stuffed Salmon

Preparation time: 10 minutes
Cooking time: 20 minutes
Servings: 2

Ingredients:
- 2 skinless and boneless salmon fillets
- 1 tablespoon of olive oil
- 5 ounces tiger shrimp
- 6 mushrooms
- 3 green onions
- 2 cups of spinach
- ¼ cup of macadamia nuts
- Salt and black pepper to taste

Instructions:
Heat up a pan with half of the oil over medium high heat, add mushrooms, onions, salt and pepper, stir and cook for 4 minutes. Add macadamia nuts, spinach and shrimp, stir, cook for 3 minutes and take off heat. Make an incision lengthwise in each salmon fillet, season with salt and pepper, divide spinach and shrimp mix into incisions and rub with the rest of the olive oil. Place in your air fryer's basket and cook at 360 degrees F and cook for 10 minutes, flipping halfway. Divide stuffed salmon on plates and serve.

Nutritional Values:
Calories 162, Fats 15g, Carbohydrates 4g, Proteins 9g, Sugar 2g

3. Mustard Salmon

Preparation time: 10 minutes
Cooking time: 10 minutes
Servings: 1

Ingredients:
- 1 big boneless salmon fillet
- Salt and black pepper to taste
- 2 tablespoons of mustard
- 1 tablespoon of coconut oil
- 1 tablespoon of maple extract

Instructions:
In a bowl, mix maple extract with mustard, whisk well, season salmon with salt and pepper and brush salmon with this mix. Spray some cooking spray over fish, place in your air fryer and cook at 370 degrees F for 10 minutes, flipping halfway. Serve with a tasty side salad.

Nutritional Values:
Calories 241, Fats 19g, Carbohydrates 5g, Proteins 7g, Sugar 4g

4. Flavored Jamaican Salmon

Preparation time: 10 minutes
Cooking time: 10 minutes
Servings: 4

Ingredients:
- 2 teaspoons of sriracha sauce
- 4 teaspoons of sugar
- 3 scallions
- Salt and black pepper to taste
- 2 teaspoons of olive oil
- 4 teaspoons of apple cider vinegar
- 3 teaspoons of avocado oil
- 4 medium salmon fillets
- 4 cups of baby arugula
- 2 cups of cabbage
- 1 and half teaspoon Jamaican jerk seasoning
- ¼ cup of toasted pepitas
- 2 cups of radish

Instructions:
In a bowl, mix sriracha with sugar, whisk and transfer 2 teaspoons to another bowl. Combine 2 teaspoons sriracha mix with the avocado oil, olive oil, vinegar, salt and pepper and whisk well. Sprinkle jerk seasoning over salmon, rub with sriracha and sugar mix and season with salt and pepper. Transfer to your air fryer and cook at 360 degrees F for 10 minutes, flipping once. In a bowl, mix radishes with cabbage, arugula, salt, pepper, sriracha and vinegar mix and toss well. Divide salmon and radish mix on plates, sprinkle pepitas and scallions on top and serve.

Nutritional Values:
Calories 70, Fats 20g, Carbohydrates 10g, Proteins 13g Sugar 9g

5. Swordfish and Mango Salsa

Preparation time: 10 minutes
Cooking time: 6 minutes
Servings: 2

Ingredients:
- 2 medium swordfish steaks
- Salt and black pepper to taste
- 2 teaspoons of avocado oil
- 1 tablespoon of cilantro
- 1 mango
- 1 avocado
- A pinch of cumin
- A pinch of onion powder
- A pinch of garlic powder
- 1 orange
- Half tablespoon balsamic vinegar

Instructions:
Season fish steaks with salt, pepper, garlic powder, onion powder and cumin and rub with half of the oil, place in your air fryer and cook at 360 degrees F for 6 minutes, flipping halfway. Meanwhile, in a bowl, mix avocado with mango, cilantro, balsamic vinegar, salt, pepper and the rest of the oil and stir well. Divide fish on plates, top with mango salsa and serve with orange slices on the side.

Nutritional Values:
Calories 200, Fats 16g, Carbohydrates 4g, Proteins 13g Sugar 10g

6. Salmon and Orange Marmalade

Preparation time: 10 minutes
Cooking time: 15 minutes
Servings: 4

Ingredients:
- 1 pound boneless and cubed wild salmon
- 2 lemons
- ¼ cup of balsamic vinegar
- ¼ cup of orange juice
- 1/3 cup of orange marmalade
- A pinch of salt and black pepper

Instructions:
Heat up a pot with the vinegar over medium heat, add marmalade and orange juice, stir, bring to a simmer, cook for 1 minute and take off heat. Thread salmon cubes and lemon slices on skewers, season with salt and black pepper, brush them with half of the orange marmalade mix, arrange in your air fryer's basket and cook at 360 degrees F for 3 minutes on each side. Brush skewers with the rest of the vinegar mix, divide among plates and serve right away with a side salad.

Nutritional Values:
Calories 60, Fats 11g, Carbohydrates 4g, Proteins 7g Sugar 6g

7. Chili Salmon

Preparation time: 10 minutes
Cooking time: 15 minutes
Servings: 12

Ingredients:
- 1 and ¼ cups coconut
- 1 pound salmon
- 1/3 cup of flour
- A pinch of salt and black pepper
- 1 egg
- 2 tablespoons of olive oil
- ¼ cup of water
- 4 red chilies
- 3 garlic cloves
- ¼ cup of balsamic vinegar
- ½ cup of honey

Instructions:
In a bowl, mix flour with a pinch of salt and stir. In another bowl, mix egg with black pepper and whisk. Put coconut in a third bowl. Dip salmon cubes in flour, egg and coconut, put them in your air fryer's basket, cook at 370 degrees F for 8 minutes, shaking halfway and divide among plates. Heat up a pan with the water over medium high heat, add chilies, cloves, vinegar and honey, stir very well, bring to a boil, simmer for a couple of minutes, drizzle over salmon and serve.

Nutritional Values:
Calories 60, Fats 16g, Carbohydrates 6g, Proteins 8g Sugar 4g

8. Salmon and Lemon Relish

Preparation time: 10 minutes
Cooking time: 30 minutes
Servings: 2

Ingredients:
- 2 salmon fillets
- Salt and black pepper to taste
- 1 tablespoon of oil

For Relish:
- 1 tablespoon of lemon juice
- 1 shallot
- 1 Meyer lemon
- 2 tablespoons of parsley
- ¼ cup of oil

Instructions:
Season salmon with salt and pepper, rub with 1 tablespoon oil, place in your air fryer's basket and cook at 320 degrees F for 20 minutes, flipping the fish halfway. Meanwhile, in a bowl, mix shallot with the lemon juice, a pinch of salt and black pepper, stir and leave aside for 10 minutes. The marinated shallots are combined with lime wedges, salt, pepper, parsley, and a quarter cup of oil in a separate bowl. Serve the salmon with the lemon relish on separate dishes.

Nutritional Values:
Calories 125, Fats 20g, Carbohydrates 11g, Proteins 14g, Sugar 7g

9. Salmon and Avocado Sauce

Preparation time: 10 minutes
Cooking time: 10 minutes
Servings: 4

Ingredients:
- 1 avocado
- 4 salmon fillets
- ¼ cup of cilantro
- 1/3 cup of coconut milk
- 1 tablespoon of lime juice
- 1 tablespoon of lime zest
- 1 teaspoon of onion powder
- 1 teaspoon of garlic powder
- Salt and black pepper to taste

Instructions:
Season salmon fillets with salt, black pepper and lime zest, rub well, put in your air fryer, cook at 350 degrees F for 9 minutes, flipping once and divide among plates. In your food processor, mix avocado with cilantro, garlic powder, onion powder, lime juice, salt, pepper and coconut milk, blend well, drizzle over salmon and serve right away.

Nutritional Values:
Calories 214, Fats 15g, Carbohydrates 9g, Proteins 5g, Sugar 4g.

10. Crusted Salmon

Preparation time: 10 minutes
Cooking time: 10 minutes
Servings: 4

Ingredients:
- 1 cup of pistachios
- 4 salmon fillets
- ¼ cup of lemon juice
- 2 tablespoons of honey
- 1 teaspoon of dill
- Salt and black pepper to taste
- 1 tablespoon of mustard

Instructions:
In a bowl, mix pistachios with mustard, honey, lemon juice, salt, black pepper and dill, whisk and spread over salmon. Put in your air fryer and cook at 350 degrees F for 10 minutes. Divide among plates and serve with a side salad.

Nutritional Values:
Calories 221, Fats 13g, Carbohydrates 6g, Proteins 9g, Sugar 5g

11. Stuffed Calamari

Preparation time: 10 minutes
Cooking time: 25 minutes
Servings: 4

Ingredients:
- 4 big calamari
- 2 tablespoons of parsley
- 5 ounces kale
- 2 garlic cloves
- 1 red bell pepper
- 1 tablespoon of oil
- 2 ounces canned tomato puree
- 1 yellow onion
- Salt and black pepper to taste

Instructions:
Heat up a pan with the oil over medium heat, add onion and garlic, stir and cook for 2 minutes. Add pepper, calamari tentacles, kale, salt and pepper and other ingredients, stir, cook for 10 minutes and take off heat. Stir and cook for 3 minutes. Stuff calamari tubes with this mix, secure with toothpicks, put in your air fryer and cook at 360 degrees F for 20 minutes. Divide calamari on plates, sprinkle parsley all over and serve.

Nutritional Values:
Calories 300, Fats 12g, Carbohydrates 3g, Proteins 8g, Sugar 4g

12. Salmon and Chives Vinaigrette

Preparation time: 10 minutes
Cooking time: 12 minutes
Servings: 4

Ingredients:
- 2 tablespoons of dill
- 4 salmon fillets
- 2 tablespoons of chives
- 1/3 cup of maple syrup
- 1 tablespoon of oil
- 3 tablespoons of balsamic vinegar
- Salt and black pepper to taste

Instructions:
Season fish with salt and pepper, rub with the oil, place in your air fryer and cook at 350 degrees F for 8 minutes, flipping once. Heat up a small pot with the vinegar over medium heat, add maple syrup, chives and dill, stir and cook for 3 minutes. Divide fish on plates and serve with chives vinaigrette on top.

Nutritional Values:
Calories 211, Fats 21g, Carbohydrates 7g, Proteins 13g, Sugar 5g

13. Roasted Cod and Prosciutto

Preparation time: 10 minutes
Cooking time: 10 minutes
Servings: 4

Ingredients:
- 1 tablespoon parsley
- 4 medium cod filets
- ¼ cup of butter
- 2 garlic cloves
- 2 tablespoons of lemon juice
- 3 tablespoons of prosciutto
- 1 teaspoon of Dijon mustard
- 1 shallot
- Salt and black pepper to taste

Instructions:
In a bowl, mix mustard with butter, garlic, parsley, shallot, lemon juice, prosciutto, salt and pepper and whisk well. Season fish with salt and pepper, spread prosciutto mix all over, put in your air fryer and cook at 390 degrees F for 10 minutes. Divide among plates and serve.

Nutritional Values:
Calories 231, Fats 33g, Carbohydrates 14g, Proteins 20g, Sugar 9g

14. Halibut and Sun-Dried Tomatoes Mix

Preparation time: 10 minutes
Cooking time: 10 minutes
Servings: 2

Ingredients:
- 2 medium halibut fillets
- 2 garlic cloves
- 2 teaspoons of oil
- Salt and black pepper to taste
- 6 sun dried tomatoes
- 2 small red onions
- 1 fennel bulb
- 9 black olives

- 4 rosemary springs
- Half teaspoon of red pepper flakes

Instructions:
Season fish with salt, pepper, rub with garlic and oil and put in a heat proof dish that fits your air fryer. Add onion slices, sun dried tomatoes, fennel, olives, rosemary and sprinkle pepper flakes, transfer to your air fryer and cook at 380 degrees F for 10 minutes. Divide fish and veggies on plates and serve.

Nutritional Values:
Calories 121, Fats 19g, Carbohydrates 3g, Proteins 13g, Sugar 10g

15. Beet, Tomato and Goat Cheese Mix

Preparation time: 30 minutes
Cooking time: 14 minutes
Servings: 8

Ingredients:
- 8 small beets
- 1 red onion
- 4 ounces goat cheese
- 1 tablespoon of balsamic vinegar
- Salt and black pepper to taste
- 2 tablespoons of sugar
- 1-pint mixed cherry tomatoes
- 2 ounces pecans
- 2 tablespoons of oil

Instructions:
Put beets in your air fryer, season them with salt and pepper, and cook at 350 degrees F for 14 minutes and transfer to a salad bowl. Add onion, cherry tomatoes and pecans and toss. In another bowl, mix vinegar with sugar and oil, whisk well until sugar dissolves and add to salad. Also add goat cheese, toss and serve.

Nutritional Values:
Calories 214, Fats 40g, Carbohydrates 12g, Proteins 24g, Sugar 11g

16. Broccoli Salad

Preparation time: 10 minutes
Cooking time: 8 minutes
Servings: 4

Ingredients:
- 1 broccoli head
- 1 tablespoon of peanut oil
- 6 garlic cloves
- 1 tablespoon of Chinese rice wine vinegar
- Salt and black pepper to taste

Instructions:
In a bowl, mix broccoli with salt, pepper and half of the oil, toss, transfer to your air fryer and cook at 350 degrees F for 8 minutes, shaking the fryer halfway. Put the broccoli in a salad dish and add the rest of the peanut oil, the garlic, and the rice vinegar. Toss everything up thoroughly and serve.

Nutritional Values:
Calories 573, Carbohydrates 5g, Protein 31g, Fat 48g, Sugar 8g

17. Brussels sprouts and Tomatoes Mix

Preparation time: 5 minutes
Cooking time: 10 minutes
Servings: 4

Ingredients:
- 1 pound Brussels sprouts
- Salt and black pepper to taste
- 6 cherry tomatoes
- ¼ cup of green onions
- 1 tablespoon of oil

Instructions:
Season Brussels sprouts with salt and pepper, put them in your air fryer and cook at 350 degrees F for 10 minutes. Transfer them to a bowl, add salt, pepper, cherry tomatoes, green onions and oil, toss well and serve.

Nutritional Values:
Calories 421, Carbohydrates 3g, Protein 22g, Fat 35g, Sugar 6g

18. Brussels sprouts and Butter Sauce

Preparation time: 4 minutes
Cooking time: 10 minutes
Servings: 4

Ingredients:
- 1 pound Brussels sprouts
- Salt and black pepper to taste
- Half cup of cooked bacon
- 1 tablespoon of mustard
- 1 tablespoon of butter
- 2 tablespoons of dill

Instructions:
Put Brussels sprouts in your air fryer and cook them at 350 degrees F for 10 minutes. Heat up a pan with the butter over medium high heat, add bacon, mustard and dill and whisk well. Divide Brussels sprouts on plates, drizzle butter sauce all over and serve.

Nutritional Values:
Calories 157, Carbohydrates 5g, Protein 6g, Fat 14g, Sugar 5g

19. Cheesy Brussels sprouts

Preparation time: 10 minutes
Cooking time: 8 minutes
Servings: 4

Ingredients:
- 1 pound Brussels sprouts
- Juice of 1 lemon
- Salt and black pepper to taste
- 2 tablespoons of butter
- 3 tablespoons of parmesan

Instructions:

Put Brussels sprouts in your air fryer, cook them at 350 degrees F for 8 minutes and transfer them to a bowl. Heat up a pan with the butter over medium heat, add lemon juice, salt and pepper, whisk well and add to Brussels sprouts. Add parmesan, toss until parmesan melts and serve.

Nutritional Values:

Calories 373, Carbohydrates 6g, Protein 26g, Fat 25g, Sugar 4g

20. Spicy Cabbage

Preparation time: 10 minutes
Cooking time: 8 minutes
Servings: 4

Ingredients:

- 1 cabbage
- 1 tablespoon of sesame seed oil
- 1 carrot
- ¼ cup of apple cider vinegar
- ¼ cups of apple juice
- Half teaspoon of cayenne pepper
- 1 teaspoon of red pepper flakes

Instructions:

In a pan that fits your air fryer, combine cabbage with oil, carrot, vinegar, apple juice, cayenne and pepper flakes, and toss, introduce in preheated air fryer and cook at 350 degrees F for 8 minutes. Divide cabbage mix on plates and serve.

Nutritional Values:

Calories 320, Carbohydrates 4g, Protein 22g, Fat 23g, Sugar 18g

21. Tasty Lamb Ribs

Preparation time: 15 minutes
Cooking time: 40 minutes
Servings: 8

Ingredients:

- 8 lamb ribs
- 4 garlic cloves
- 2 carrots
- 2 cups of veggie stock
- 1 tablespoon of rosemary
- 2 tablespoons of oil
- Salt and black pepper to taste
- 3 tablespoons of white flour

Instructions:

Season lamb ribs with salt and pepper, rub with oil and garlic, put in preheated air fryer and cook at 360 degrees F for 10 minutes. In a heat proof dish that fits your fryer, mix stock with flour and whisk well. Add rosemary, carrots and lamb ribs, place in your air fryer and cook at 350 degrees F for 30 minutes. Divide lamb mix on plates and serve hot.

Nutritional Values:

Calories 441, Carbohydrates 3g, Protein 23g, Fat 34g, Sugar 7g

22. Oriental Air Fried Lamb

Preparation time: 10 minutes
Cooking time: 42 minutes
Servings: 8

Ingredients:
- 2 and half pound's lamb shoulder
- 3 tablespoons of honey
- 3 ounces almonds
- 9 ounces plumps
- 8 ounces veggie stock
- 2 yellow onions
- 2 garlic cloves
- Salt and black pepper to tastes
- 1 teaspoon of cumin powder
- 1 teaspoon of turmeric powder
- 1 teaspoon of ginger powder
- 1 teaspoon of cinnamon powder
- 3 tablespoons of olive oil

Instructions:
In a bowl, mix cinnamon powder with ginger, cumin, turmeric, garlic, olive oil and lamb, toss to coat, place in your preheated air fryer and cook at 350 degrees F for 8 minutes. Transfer meat to a dish that fits your air fryer, add onions, stock, honey and plums, stir, introduce in your air fryer and cook at 350 degrees F for 35 minutes. Divide everything on plates and serve with almond sprinkled on top.

Nutritional Values:
Calories 194, Carbohydrates 2g, Protein 8g, Fat 17g, Sugar 5g

23. Short Ribs and Special Sauce

Preparation time: 10 minutes
Cooking time: 36 minutes
Servings: 4

Ingredients:
- 2 green onions
- 1 teaspoon of vegetable oil
- 3 garlic cloves
- 3 ginger slices
- 4 pounds short ribs
- Half cup of water
- Half cup of soy sauce
- ¼ cup of rice wine
- ¼ cup of pear juice
- 2 teaspoons of sesame oil

Instructions:
Heat up a pan that fits your air fryer with the oil over medium heat, add green onions, ginger and garlic, stir and cook for 1 minute. Add ribs, water, wine, soy sauce, sesame oil and pear juice, stir, introduce in your air fryer and cook at 350 degrees F for 35 minutes. Divide ribs and sauce on plates and serve.

Nutritional Values:
Calories 80, Carbohydrates 1g, Protein 6g, Fat 4g

24. Short Ribs and Beer Sauce

Preparation time: 15 minutes
Cooking time: 45 minutes
Servings: 6

Ingredients:
- 4 pounds short ribs
- 1 yellow onion
- Salt and black pepper to taste
- ¼ cup of tomato paste
- 1 cup of dark beer
- 1 cup of chicken stock
- 1 bay leaf
- 6 thyme springs
- 1 Portobello mushroom

Instructions:
Heat up a pan that fits your air fryer over medium heat, add tomato paste, onion, stock, beer, mushroom, bay leaves and thyme and bring to a simmer. Add ribs, introduce in your air fryer and cook at 350 degrees F for 40 minutes. Divide everything on plates and serve.

Nutritional Values:
Calories 400, Carbohydrates 9g, Protein 12g, Fat 33g, Sugar 6g

25. Sesame-Crusted Tuna with Green Beans

Prep Time: 15 minutes
Cook Time: 5 minutes
Servings: 4

Ingredients
- ¼ cup of white sesame seeds
- ¼ cup of black sesame seeds
- 4 tuna steaks
- Salt and pepper
- 1 tablespoon oil
- 1 tablespoon of coconut oil
- 2 cups of green beans

Instructions
In a wide bowl, mix together the two kinds of sesame seeds. Put some salt and pepper on the tuna. Coat the tuna with the sesame seed flour. Olive oil should be heated over high heat before being added to the tuna. Sear one side for 1-2 minutes, then flip and repeat. Take the tuna out of the pan and let it rest while you heat the coconut oil in the pan. Serve sliced tuna on top of green beans that have been fried in oil for 5 minutes.

Nutritional Values
380 calories, 19g fat, 44.5g protein, 8g carbs, 3g fiber, 5g net Carbs

26. Grilled Salmon and Zucchini with Mango Sauce

Prep Time: 5 minutes
Cook Time: 10 minutes
Servings: 4

Ingredients
- 4 boneless of salmon fillets
- 1 tablespoon of olive oil
- Salt and pepper
- 1 zucchini
- 2 tablespoons of lemon juice
- ½ cup of chopped mango
- ¼ cup of cilantro
- 1 teaspoon of lemon zest
- ½ cup of coconut milk

Instructions
Prepare a grill pan by heating it over high heat and spraying it heavily with cooking spray. Season the salmon with salt and pepper and brush it with olive oil. Sprinkle the zucchini with salt and pepper and toss it with some lemon juice. Prepare a grill for the fish and zucchini. Put everything in the oven for 5 minutes, then flip and cook for another 5 minutes. Make a sauce by blending the remaining ingredients together in a blender. Mango sauce drizzled over salmon fillets, with a side of zucchini.

Nutritional Values
350 calories, 21.5g fat, 35g protein, 8g carbs, 2g fiber, 6g net Carbs

27. Parmesan-Crusted Halibut with Asparagus

Prep Time: 10 minutes
Cook Time: 15 minutes
Servings: 4

Ingredients
- 1 pound asparagus
- 2 tablespoons of olive oil
- Salt and pepper
- ¼ cup butter
- ¼ cup of parmesan
- 2 tablespoons of almond flour
- 1 teaspoon of garlic powder
- 4 boneless of halibut fillets

Instructions
Turn the oven on to 400 degrees Fahrenheit and line a baking sheet with foil. Prepare a baking sheet by spreading the asparagus and tossing it with olive oil. Blend the butter, parmesan cheese, almond flour, garlic powder, salt, and pepper. Spread the parmesan mixture over the fillets and set them on the baking pan alongside the asparagus—ten to twelve minutes in the oven, followed by two to three minutes under the broiler.

Nutritional Values
415 calories, 26g fat, 42g protein, 6g carbs, 3g fiber, 3g net Carbs

28. Beef Stuffed Squash

Preparation time: 10 minutes
Cooking time: 40 minutes
Servings: 2

Ingredients:
- 1 spaghetti squash
- 1 pound beef
- Salt and black pepper to taste
- 3 garlic cloves
- 1 yellow onion
- 1 Portobello mushroom
- 28 ounces canned tomatoes
- 1 teaspoon of oregano
- ¼ teaspoon of cayenne pepper
- Half teaspoon of dry thyme
- 1 green bell pepper

Instructions:
Put spaghetti squash in your air fryer, cook at 350 degrees F for 20 minutes, transfer to a cutting board, and cut into halves and discard seeds. Heat up a pan over medium high heat, add meat, garlic, onion and mushroom, stir and cook until meat browns. Add salt, pepper, thyme, oregano, cayenne, tomatoes and green pepper, stir and cook for 10 minutes. Stuff squash with this beef mix, introduce in the fryer and cook at 360 degrees F for 10 minutes. Divide among plates and serve.

Nutritional Values:
Calories 584, Carbohydrates 9g, Protein 46g, Fat 41g, Sugar 12g

29. Greek Beef Meatballs Salad

Preparation time: 10 minutes
Cooking time: 10 minutes
Servings: 6

Ingredients:
- ¼ cup of milk
- 17 ounces beef
- 1 yellow onion
- 5 bread slices
- 1 egg
- ¼ cup of parsley
- Salt and black pepper to taste
- 2 garlic cloves
- ¼ cup of mint
- 2 and half teaspoons oregano
- 1 tablespoon of olive oil
- Cooking spray
- 7 ounces cherry tomatoes
- 1 cup of baby spinach
- 1 and half tablespoons of lemon juice
- 7 ounces Greek yogurt

Instructions:
Put torn bread in a bowl, add milk, soak for a few minutes, squeeze and transfer to another bowl. Add beef, egg, salt, pepper, oregano, mint, parsley, garlic and onion, stir and shape medium meatballs out of this mix. Spray them with cooking spray, place them in your air fryer and cook at 370 degrees F for 10 minutes. In a salad bowl, mix spinach with cucumber and tomato. Add meatballs, the oil, some salt, pepper, lemon juice and yogurt, toss and serve.

Nutritional Values:
Calories 95, Carbohydrates 1g, Protein 7g, Fat 7g, Sugar 14g

30. Beef Patties and Mushroom Sauce

Preparation time: 10 minutes
Cooking time: 25 minutes
Servings: 6

Ingredients:
- 2 pounds beef
- Salt and black pepper to taste
- Half teaspoon of garlic powder
- 1 tablespoon of soy sauce
- ¼ cup of beef stock
- ¾ cup of flour
- 1 tablespoon of parsley
- 1 tablespoon of onion flakes

For the sauce:
- 1 cup of yellow onion
- 2 cups of mushrooms
- 2 tablespoons of bacon Fats
- 2 tablespoons of butter
- Half teaspoon of soy sauce
- ¼ cup of sour cream
- Half cup of beef stock
- Salt and black pepper to taste

Instructions:
In a bowl, mix beef with salt, pepper, garlic powder, 1 tablespoon soy sauce, ¼ cup beef stock, flour, parsley and onion flakes, stir well, shape 6 patties, place them in your air fryer and cook at 350 degrees F for 14 minutes. Meanwhile, heat up a pan with the butter and the bacon Fats over medium heat, add mushrooms, stir and cook for 4 minutes. Add onions, stir and cook for 4 minutes more. Add ½ teaspoon soy sauce, sour cream and ½ cup stock, stir well, bring to a simmer and take off heat. Divide beef patties on plates and serve with mushroom sauce on top.

Nutritional Values: Calories 484, Carbohydrates 7g, Protein 12g, Fat 46g, Sugar 11g

31. Beef Casserole

Preparation time: 30 minutes
Cooking time: 35 minutes
Servings: 12

Ingredients:
- 1 tablespoon of olive oil
- 2 pounds beef
- 2 cups of eggplant
- Salt and black pepper to taste
- 2 teaspoons of mustard
- 2 teaspoons of gluten free Worcestershire sauce
- 28 ounces canned tomatoes
- 2 cups of mozzarella
- 16 ounces tomato sauce
- 2 tablespoons of parsley
- 1 teaspoon of oregano

Instructions:
In a bowl, mix eggplant with salt, pepper and oil and toss to coat. In another bowl, mix beef with salt, pepper, mustard and Worcestershire sauce, stir well and spread on the bottom of a pan that fits your air fryer. Add eggplant mix, tomatoes, tomato sauce, parsley, oregano and sprinkle mozzarella at the end. Introduce in your air fryer and cook at 360 degrees F for 35 minutes. Divide among plates and serve hot.

Nutritional Values:
Calories 680, Carbohydrates 8g, Protein 30g, Fat 55g, Sugar 10g

32. Lamb and Spinach Mix

Preparation time: 10 minutes
Cooking time: 35 minutes
Servings: 6

Ingredients:
- 2 tablespoons of ginger
- 2 garlic cloves
- 2 teaspoons of cardamom
- 1 red onion
- 1 pound lamb meat
- 2 teaspoons of cumin powder
- 1 teaspoon of garam masala
- Half teaspoon of chili powder
- 1 teaspoon of turmeric
- 2 teaspoons of coriander
- 1 pound spinach
- 14 ounces canned tomatoes

Instructions:
In a heat proof dish that fits your air fryer, mix lamb with spinach, tomatoes, ginger, garlic, onion, cardamom, cloves, cumin, garam masala, chili, turmeric and coriander, stir, introduce in preheated air fryer and cook at 360 degrees F for 35 minutes Divide into bowls and serve.

Nutritional Values:
Calories 680, Carbohydrates 8g, Protein 30g, Fat 55g, Sugar 8g

33. Lamb and Lemon Sauce

Preparation time: 10 minutes
Cooking time: 30 minutes
Servings: 4

Ingredients:
- 2 lamb shanks
- Salt and black pepper to taste
- 2 garlic cloves
- 4 tablespoons of olive oil
- Juice from half lemon
- Zest from half lemon
- Half teaspoon of oregano

Instructions:
Season lamb with salt, pepper, rub with garlic, put in your air fryer and cook at 350 degrees F for 30 minutes. Meanwhile, in a bowl, mix lemon juice with lemon zest, some salt and pepper, the olive oil and oregano and whisk very well. Shred lamb, discard bone, divide among plates, drizzle the lemon dressing all over and serve.

Nutritional Values:
Calories 290, Carbohydrates 4g, Protein 15g, Fat 24g, Sugar 7g

34. Lamb and Green Pesto

Preparation time: 1 hour
Cooking time: 45 minutes
Servings: 4

Ingredients:
- 1 cup of parsley
- 1 cup of mint
- 1 small yellow onion
- 1/3 cup of pistachios
- 1 teaspoon of lemon zest
- 5 tablespoons of olive oil
- Salt and black pepper to taste
- 2 pounds lamb riblets
- Half onion
- 5 garlic cloves
- Juice from 1 orange

Instructions:
In your food processor, mix parsley with mint, onion, pistachios, lemon zest, salt, pepper and oil and blend very well. Rub lamb with this mix, place in a bowl, cover and leave in the fridge for 1 hour. Transfer lamb to a baking dish that fits your air fryer, also add garlic, drizzle orange juice and cook in your air fryer at 300 degrees F for 45 minutes. Divide lamb on plates and serve.

Nutritional Values:
Calories 120, Carbohydrates 2g, Protein 7g, Fat 9g, Sugar 2g

35. Burgundy Beef Mix

Preparation time: 10 minutes
Cooking time: 1 hour
Servings: 7

Ingredients:
- 2 pounds beef chuck roast
- 15 ounces canned tomatoes
- 4 carrots
- Salt and black pepper to taste
- Half pounds mushroom
- 2 celery ribs
- 2 yellow onions
- 1 cup of beef stock
- 1 tablespoon of thyme
- Half teaspoon of mustard powder
- 3 tablespoons of almond flour
- 1 cup of water

Instructions:
Heat up a heat proof pot that fits your air fryer over medium high heat, add beef, stir and brown them for a couple of minutes. Add tomatoes, mushrooms, onions, carrots, celery, salt, pepper mustard, stock and thyme and stir. In a bowl mix water with flour, stir well, add this to the pot, toss, introduce in your air fryer and cook at 300 degrees F for 1 hour. Divide into bowls and serve.

Nutritional Values:
Calories 108, Carbohydrates 4g, Protein 7g, Fat 6g, Sugar 4g

Chapter 7: Appetizers and Snacks

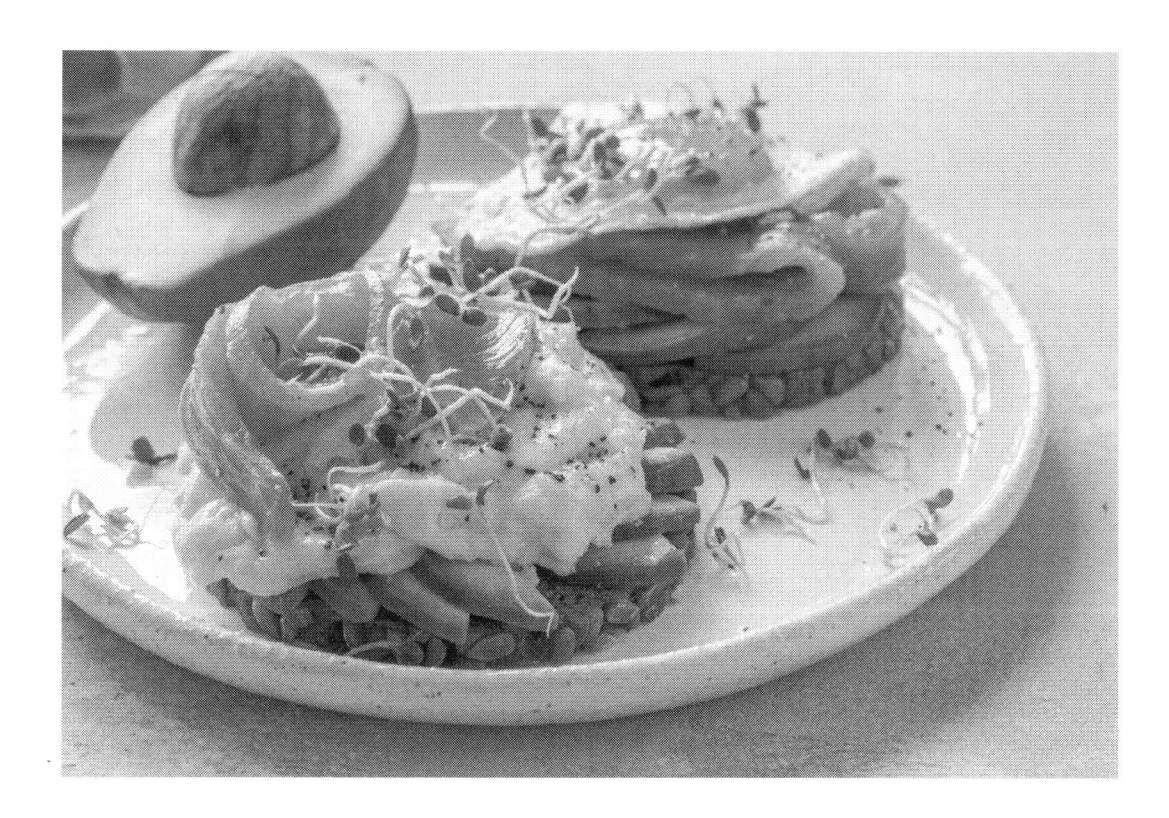

1. Mushrooms and Sour Cream

Preparation time: 10 minutes
Cooking time: 10 minutes
Servings: 6

Ingredients:
- 2 bacon strips
- 1 onion
- 1 bell pepper
- 24 mushrooms
- 1 carrot
- Half cup of cream
- 1 cup of cheese
- Salt and black pepper to taste

Instructions:

Heat up a pan over medium high heat, add bacon, onion, bell pepper and carrot, stir and cook for 1 minute. Add salt, pepper and sour cream, stir cook for 1 minute more, take off heat and cool down. Stuff mushrooms with this mix, sprinkle cheese on top and cook at 360 degrees F for 8 minutes. Divide among plates and serve as a side dish.

Nutritional Values:
Calories 211, Fats 14g, Carbohydrates 8g, Proteins 3g, Sugar 2g

2. Eggplant Fries

Preparation time: 10 minutes
Cooking time: 5 minutes
Servings: 4

Ingredients:
- Cooking spray
- 1 eggplant
- 2 tablespoons of milk
- 1 egg
- 2 cups of bread crumbs
- Half cup of cheese
- A pinch of salt and black pepper to taste

Instructions:
In a bowl, mix egg with milk, salt and pepper and whisk well. In another bowl, mix panko with cheese and stir. Dip eggplant fries in egg mix, then coat in panko mix, place them in your air fryer greased with cooking spray and cook at 400 degrees F for 5 minutes. Divide among plates and serve as a side dish.

Nutritional Values: Calories 162, Fats 15g, Carbohydrates 4g, Proteins 9g, Sugar 2g

3. Buffalo Cauliflower Snack

Preparation time: 10 minutes
Cooking time: 15 minutes
Servings: 4

Ingredients:
- 4 cups of cauliflower florets
- 1 cup of bread crumbs
- ¼ cup of butter
- ¼ cup of buffalo sauce
- Mayonnaise for serving

Instructions:
In a bowl, mix buffalo sauce with butter and whisk well. Dip cauliflower florets in this mix and coat them in panko bread crumbs. Place them in your air fryer's basket and cook at 350 degrees F for 15 minutes. Arrange them on a platter and serve with mayo on the side.

Nutritional Values: Calories 241, Fats 19g, Carbohydrates 5g, Proteins 7g, Sugar 4g

4. Banana Snack

Preparation time: 10 minutes
Cooking time: 5 minutes
Servings: 8

Ingredients:
- 16 baking cups of crust
- ¼ cup of peanut butter
- ¾ cups of chocolate chips
- 1 banana
- 1 tablespoon of oil

Instructions:
Put chocolate chips in a small pot, heat up over low heat, stir until it melts and take off heat. In a bowl, mix peanut butter with coconut oil and whisk well. Spoon 1 teaspoon chocolate mix in a cup, add 1 banana slice and top with 1 teaspoon butter mix. Repeat with the rest of the cups, place them all into a dish that fits your air fryer, cook at 320 degrees F for 5 minutes, transfer to a freezer and keep there until you serve them as a snack.

Nutritional Values: Calories 70, Fats 20g, Carbohydrates 10g, Proteins 13g Sugar 9g

5. Mexican Apple Snack

Preparation time: 10 minutes
Cooking time: 5 minutes
Servings: 4

Ingredients:
- 3 big apples
- 2 teaspoons of lemon juice
- ¼ cup of pecans
- Half cup of chocolate chips
- Half cup of clean caramel sauce

Instructions:
In a bowl, mix apples with lemon juice, stir and transfer to a pan that fits your air fryer. Add chocolate chips, pecans, drizzle the caramel sauce, toss, introduce in your air fryer and cook at 320 degrees F for 5 minutes. Toss gently, divide into small bowls and serve right away as a snack.

Nutritional Values:
Calories 200, Fats 16g, Carbohydrates 4g, Proteins 13g Sugar 10g

6. Shrimp Muffins

Preparation time: 10 minutes
Cooking time: 26 minutes
Servings: 6

Ingredients:
- 1 spaghetti squash
- 2 tablespoons of mayonnaise
- 1 cup of mozzarella
- 8 ounces of shrimp
- 1 and a half cups of panko
- 1 teaspoons of parsley flakes
- 1 garlic clove
- Salt and black pepper to taste
- Cooking spray

Instructions:
Put squash halves in your air fryer, cook at 350 degrees F for 16 minutes, leave aside to cool down and scrape flesh into a bowl. Add salt, pepper, parsley flakes, panko, shrimp, mayo and mozzarella and stir well. Spray a muffin tray that fits your air fryer with cooking spray and divide squash and shrimp mix in each cup. Introduce in the fryer and cook at 360 degrees F for 10 minutes. Arrange muffins on a platter and serve as a snack.

Nutritional Values:
Calories 60, Fats 11g, Carbohydrates 4g, Proteins 7g Sugar 6g

7. Zucchini Cakes

Preparation time: 10 minutes
Cooking time: 12 minutes
Servings: 12

Ingredients:
- Cooking spray
- Half cup of dill
- 1 egg
- Half cup of wheat flour
- Salt and black pepper to taste
- 1 onion
- 2 garlic cloves
- 3 zucchinis

Instructions:
In a bowl, mix zucchinis with garlic, onion, flour, salt, pepper, egg and dill, stir well, shape small patties out of this mix, spray them with cooking spray, place them in your air fryer's basket and cook at 370 degrees F for 6 minutes on each side. Serve them as a snack right away.

Nutritional Values:
Calories 60, Fats 16g, Carbohydrates 6g, Proteins 8g Sugar 4g

8. Cauliflower Cakes

Preparation time: 10 minutes
Cooking time: 10 minutes
Servings: 6

Ingredients:
- 3 and a half cups of cauliflower rice
- 2 eggs
- ¼ cup of flour
- Half cup of parmesan
- Salt and black pepper to taste
- Cooking spray

Instructions:
In a bowl, mix cauliflower rice with salt and pepper, stir and squeeze excess water. Transfer cauliflower to another bowl, add eggs, salt, pepper, flour and parmesan, stir really well and shape your cakes. Grease your air fryer with cooking spray, heat it up at 400 degrees, add cauliflower cakes and cook them for 10 minutes flipping them halfway. Divide cakes on plates and serve as a side dish.

Nutritional Values:
Calories 125, Fats 20g, Carbohydrates 11g, Proteins 14g, Sugar 7g

9. Creamy Brussels sprouts

Preparation time: 10 minutes
Cooking time: 25 minutes
Servings: 8

Ingredients:
- 3 pounds of Brussels
- A drizzle of oil
- 1 pound of bacon
- Salt and black pepper to taste
- 4 tablespoons of butter
- 3 shallots
- 1 cup of milk
- 2 cups of heavy cream
- ¼ teaspoon of nutmeg
- 3 tablespoons of horseradish

Instructions:
Preheated you air fryer at 370 degrees F, add oil, bacon, salt and pepper and Brussels sprouts and toss. Add butter, shallots, heavy cream, milk, nutmeg and horseradish, toss again and cook for 25 minutes. Divide among plates and serve as a side dish.

Nutritional Values:
Calories 214, Fats 15g, Carbohydrates 9g, Proteins 5g, Sugar 4g.

10. Cheddar Biscuits

Preparation time: 10 minutes
Cooking time: 20 minutes
Servings: 8

Ingredients:
- 2 and quarter cups of flour
- Half cup of butter
- 1 tablespoon of melted butter
- 2 tablespoons of sugar
- Half cup of cheese
- 1 and 1/3 cups of buttermilk
- 1 cup of flour

Instructions:
In a bowl, mix self-rising flour with ½ cup butter, sugar, cheddar cheese and buttermilk and stir until you obtain a dough. Spread 1 cup flour on a working surface, roll dough, flatten it, cut 8 circles with a cookie cutter and coat them with flour. Line your air fryer's basket with tin foil, add biscuits, brush them with melted butter and cook them at 380 degrees F for 20 minutes. Divide among plates and serve as a side.

Nutritional Values:
Calories 221, Fats 13g, Carbohydrates 6g, Proteins 9g, Sugar 5g

11. Beef Jerky Snack

Preparation time: 2 hours
Cooking time: 1 hour and 30 minutes
Servings: 6

Ingredients:
- 2 cups of soy sauce
- Half cup of Worcestershire sauce
- 2 tablespoons of black peppercorns
- 2 tablespoons of black pepper
- 2 pounds of beef round

Instructions:
Soy sauce, black peppercorns, black pepper, and Worcestershire sauce are mixed together and whisked until smooth. Add beef slices, toss to coat and leave aside in the fridge for 6 hours. Introduce beef rounds in your air fryer and cook them at 370 degrees F for 1 hour and 30 minutes. Transfer to a bowl and serve cold.

Nutritional Values:
Calories 300, Fats 12g, Carbohydrates 3g, Proteins 8g, Sugar 4g

12. Honey Party Wings

Preparation time: 1 hour and 10 minutes
Cooking time: 12 minutes
Servings: 8

Ingredients:
- 16 wings of chicken
- 2 tablespoons of soy sauce
- 2 tablespoons of honey
- Salt and black pepper to taste
- 2 tablespoons of lime juice

Instructions:
Soy sauce, honey, salt, pepper, and lime juice are tossed with chicken wings and stored in the refrigerator for an hour. Transfer chicken wings to your air fryer and cook them at 360 degrees F for 12 minutes, flipping them halfway. Arrange them on a platter and serve as an appetizer.

Nutritional Values:
Calories 211, Fats 21g, Carbohydrates 7g, Proteins 13g, Sugar 5g

13. Salmon Party Patties

Preparation time: 10 minutes
Cooking time: 22 minutes
Servings: 4

Ingredients:
- 3 potatoes
- 1 big salmon fillet
- 2 tablespoons of parsley
- 2 tablespoon dill
- Salt and black pepper to taste
- 1 egg
- 2 tablespoons of bread crumbs
- Cooking spray

Instructions:
Place salmon in your air fryer's basket and cook for 10 minutes at 360 degrees F. Transfer salmon to a cutting board, cool it down, flake it and put it in a bowl. Add mashed potatoes, salt, pepper, dill, parsley, egg and bread crumbs, stir well and shape 8 patties out of this mix. Place salmon patties in your air fryer's basket, spry them with cooking oil, cook at 360 degrees F for 12 minutes, flipping them halfway, transfer them to a platter and serve as an appetizer.

Nutritional Values:
Calories 231, Fats 33g, Carbohydrates 14g, Proteins 20g, Sugar 9g

14. Banana Chips

Preparation time: 10 minutes
Cooking time: 15 minutes
Servings: 4

Ingredients:
- 4 bananas
- A pinch of salt
- Half teaspoon of turmeric powder
- Half teaspoon of chaat masala
- 1 teaspoon of olive oil

Instructions:
In a bowl, mix banana slices with salt, turmeric, chaat masala and oil, toss and leave aside for 10 minutes. Transfer banana slices to your preheated air fryer at 360 degrees F and cook them for 15 minutes flipping them once. Serve as a snack.

Nutritional Values:
Calories 121, Fats 19g, Carbohydrates 3g, Proteins 13g, Sugar 10g

15. Spring Rolls

Preparation time: 10 minutes
Cooking time: 25 minutes
Servings: 8

Ingredients:
- 2 cups of green cabbage
- 2 onions
- 1 carrot
- Half chili peppers
- 1 tablespoon of ginger
- 3 garlic cloves
- 1 teaspoon sugar
- Salt and black pepper to taste
- 1 teaspoon of soy sauce
- 2 tablespoons of olive oil
- 10 spring roll sheets
- 2 tablespoons of corn flour
- 2 tablespoons of water

Instructions:
Heat up a pan with the oil over medium heat, add cabbage, onions, carrots, chili pepper, ginger, garlic, sugar, salt, pepper and soy sauce, stir well, cook for 2-3 minutes, take off heat and cool down. Cut spring roll sheets in squares, divide cabbage mix on each and roll them. In a bowl, mix corn flour with water, stir well and seal spring rolls with this mix. Place spring rolls in your air fryer's basket and cook them at 360 degrees F for 10 minutes. Flip roll and cook them for 10 minutes more. Arrange on a platter and serve them as an appetizer.

Nutritional Values:
Calories 214, Fats 40g, Carbohydrates 12g, Proteins 24g, Sugar 11g

16. Crispy Radish Chips

Preparation time: 10 minutes
Cooking time: 10 minutes
Servings: 4

Ingredients:
- Cooking spray
- 15 radishes
- Salt and black pepper to taste
- 1 tablespoon of chives

Instructions:
Arrange radish slices in your air fryer's basket, spray them with cooking oil, season with salt and black pepper to the taste, cook them at 350 degrees F for 10 minutes, flipping them halfway, transfer to bowls and serve with chives sprinkled on top.

Nutritional Values:
Calories 221, Fats 13g, Carbohydrates 6g, Proteins 9g, Sugar 5g

17. Tortilla Chips

Preparation time: 10 minutes
Cooking time: 6 minutes
Servings: 4

Ingredients:
- 8 corns of tortillas
- Salt and black pepper to taste
- 1 tablespoon of olive oil
- A pinch of garlic powder
- A pinch of paprika

Instructions:
In a bowl, mix tortilla chips with oil, add salt, pepper, garlic powder and paprika, toss well, place them in your air fryer's basket and cook them at 400 degrees F for 6 minutes. Serve them as a side for a fish dish.

Nutritional Values:
Calories 125, Fats 20g, Carbohydrates 11g, Proteins 14g, Sugar 7g

18. Zucchini Croquettes

Preparation time: 10 minutes
Cooking time: 10 minutes
Servings: 4

Ingredients:
- 1 carrot
- 1 zucchini
- 2 slices of bread
- 1 egg
- Salt and black pepper to taste
- Half teaspoon of paprika
- 1 teaspoon of garlic
- 2 tablespoons of cheese
- 1 tablespoon of corn flour

Instructions:

Put zucchini in a bowl, add salt, leave aside for 10 minutes, squeeze excess water and transfer them to another bowl. Add carrots, salt, pepper, paprika, garlic, flour, parmesan, egg and bread crumbs, stir well, shape 8 croquettes, place them in your air fryer and cook at 360 degrees F for 10 minutes. Divide among plates and serve as a side dish

Nutritional Values:

Calories 60, Fats 26g, Carbohydrates 7g, Proteins 18g Sugar 5g

19. Chickpeas Snack

Preparation time: 10 minutes
Cooking time: 10 minutes
Servings: 4

Ingredients:

- 15 ounces of canned chickpeas
- Half teaspoon of cumin
- 1 tablespoon of oil
- 1 teaspoon of smoked paprika
- Salt and black pepper to taste

Instructions:

In a bowl, mix chickpeas with oil, cumin, paprika, salt and pepper, toss to coat, place them in your fryer's basket and cook at 390 degrees F for 10 minutes. Divide into bowls and serve as a snack.

Nutritional Values:

Calories 60, Fats 16g, Carbohydrates 6g, Proteins 8g Sugar 4g

20. Sausage Balls

Preparation time: 10 minutes
Cooking time: 15 minutes
Servings: 9

Ingredients:

- 4 ounces of sausage meat
- Salt and black pepper to taste
- 1 teaspoon sage
- Half teaspoon of garlic
- 1 onion
- 3 tablespoons of bread crumbs

Instructions:

In a bowl, mix sausage with salt, pepper, sage, garlic, onion and breadcrumbs, stir well and shape small balls out of this mix. Put them in your air fryer's basket, cook at 360 degrees F for 15 minutes, divide into bowls and serve as a snack.

Nutritional Values:

Calories 200, Fats 16g, Carbohydrates 4g, Proteins 13g Sugar 10g

21. Chicken Dip

Preparation time: 10 minutes
Cooking time: 25 minutes
Servings: 10

Ingredients:

- 3 tablespoons of butter
- 1 cup of yogurt
- 12 ounces of creamy cheese
- 2 cups of chicken meat
- 2 teaspoons of curry powder
- 4 scallions
- 6 ounces of Monterey jack cheese
- 1/3 cup of raisins
- ¼ cup of cilantro
- Half cup of almonds
- Salt and black pepper to taste
- Half cup of chutney

Instructions:

In a bowl mix cream cheese with yogurt and whisk using your mixer. Add curry powder, scallions, chicken meat, raisins, cheese, cilantro, salt and pepper and stir everything. Spread this into a baking dish that fist your air fryer, sprinkle almonds on top, place in your air fryer, bake at 300 degrees for 25 minutes, divide into bowls, top with chutney and serve as an appetizer.

Nutritional Values:
Calories 70, Fats 20g, Carbohydrates 10g, Proteins 13g Sugar 9g

22. Sweet Popcorn

Preparation time: 5 minutes
Cooking time: 10 minutes
Servings: 4

Ingredients:

- 2 tablespoons of corn kernels
- 2 and a half tablespoons of butter
- 2 ounces of brown sugar

Instructions:

Put corn kernels in your air fryer's pan, cook at 400 degrees F for 6 minutes, transfer them to a tray, spread and leave aside for now. Heat up a pan over low heat, add butter, melt it, add sugar and stir until it dissolves. Add popcorn, toss to coat, take off heat and spread on the tray again. Cool down, divide into bowls and serve as a snack.

Nutritional Values:
Calories 162, Fats 15g, Carbohydrates 4g, Proteins 9g, Sugar 2g

23. Apple Chips

Preparation time: 10 minutes
Cooking time: 10 minutes
Servings: 2

Ingredients:
- 1 apple
- A pinch of salt
- Half teaspoon of cinnamon powder
- 1 tablespoon of white sugar

Instructions:
In a bowl, mix apple slices with salt, sugar and cinnamon, toss, transfer to your air fryer's basket, cook for 10 minutes at 390 degrees F flipping once. Divide apple chips in bowls and serve as a snack.

Nutritional Values:
Calories 211, Fats 14g, Carbohydrates 8g, Proteins 3g, Sugar 2g

24. Bread Sticks

Preparation time: 10 minutes
Cooking time: 10 minutes
Servings: 2

Ingredients:
- 4 bread slices
- 2 eggs
- ¼ cup of milk
- 1 teaspoon of cinnamon powder
- 1 tablespoon of honey
- ¼ cup brown of sugar
- A pinch of nutmeg

Instructions:
In a bowl, mix eggs with milk, brown sugar, cinnamon, nutmeg and honey and whisk well. Dip bread sticks in this mix, place them in your air fryer's basket and cook at 360 degrees F for 10 minutes. Divide bread sticks into bowls and serve as a snack.

Nutritional Values:
Calories 214, Fats 15g, Carbohydrates 9g, Proteins 5g, Sugar 4g.

25. Crispy Shrimp

Preparation time: 10 minutes
Cooking time: 5 minutes
Servings: 4

Ingredients:
- 12 big shrimp
- 2 egg whites
- 1 cup of coconut
- 1 cup of bread crumbs
- 1 cup of flour
- Salt and black pepper to taste

Instructions:
In a bowl, mix panko with coconut and stir. Put flour, salt and pepper in a second bowl and whisk egg whites in a third one. Dip shrimp in flour, egg whites mix and coconut, place them all in your air fryer's basket, and cook at 350 degrees F for 10 minutes flipping halfway. Arrange on a platter and serve as an appetizer.

Nutritional Values:
Calories 221, Fats 13g, Carbohydrates 6g, Proteins 9g, Sugar 5g

26. Coconut Chicken Curry with Cauliflower Rice

Prep Time: 15 minutes
Cook Time: 30 minutes
Servings: 6

Ingredients
- 1 tablespoon of olive oil
- 1 onion
- 1 and ½ pounds of boneless chicken thighs
- Salt and pepper
- 1 can of coconut milk
- 1 tablespoon curry powder
- 1 and ¼ teaspoons of turmeric
- 3 cups of riced cauliflower

Instructions
Oil should be heated over medium heat in a big skillet. After around 5 minutes, the onions should be transparent and ready to be added. Add the chicken, salt, and pepper; cook for 6 to 8 minutes, tossing frequently, until browned on all sides. Add the curry powder and turmeric to the skillet once the coconut milk is poured. Reduce heat and simmer for 15–20 minutes or until bubbling and heated. In the meantime, cook the cauliflower rice in a steamer with a few tablespoons of water. Cauliflower rice should be served with curry.

Nutritional Values
430 calories, 29g fat, 33.5g protein, 9g carbs, 3.5g fiber, 5.5g net carbs

Chapter 8: Desserts

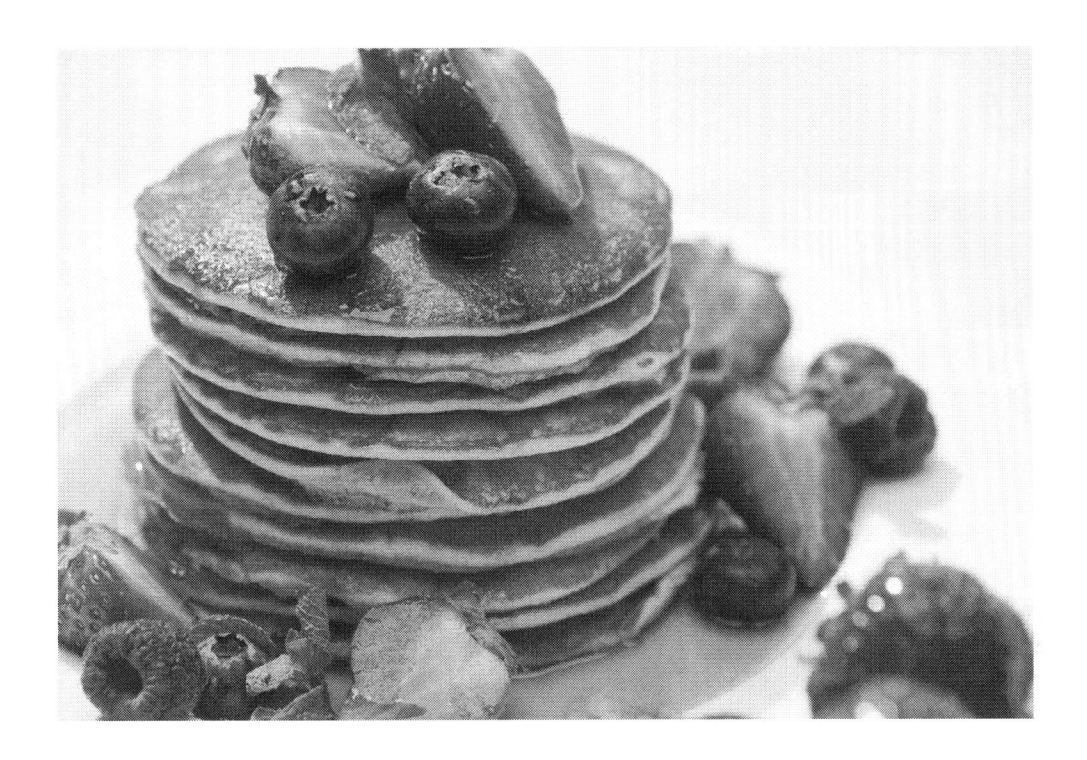

1. Almond Butter Cookie Balls
Preparation time: 5 minutes
Cooking time: 10 minutes
Serving: 10 balls

Ingredients
- 1 cup of almond butter
- 1 egg
- 1 teaspoon of vanilla extract
- 1/4 cup of low-car and sugar-free chocolate chips
- 1/4 cup of low-carb protein powder
- 1/4 cup of powdered erythritol
- 1/4 cup of shredded unsweetened coconut
- 1/2 teaspoon of cinnamon

Instructions
Combine almond butter and egg in a big basin. Vanilla, protein powder and erythritol should also be added. Add cinnamon, chocolate chips, and coconut by folding. Make one ball. Put the balls in a 6" baking pan and within the air fryer basket. The timer should be set for 10 minutes with the temperature adjusted to 320°F. Let it cool. For up to four days, keep in the refrigerator in an airtight container.

Nutritional Values
Calories: 224, Protein: 11.2g, Carbohydrates: 1.3g, Fat: 16.0g, Sugar: 1.3 g

2. Caramel Bread

Preparation time: 15 minutes
Cooking time: 12 minutes
Serving: 6

Ingredients

- 1/2 cup of low-carb vanilla protein powder
- 3/4 cup of granular erythritol, divided
- 1/2 teaspoon of baking powder
- 8 tablespoons of salted butter (melted & separated)
- 1/2 cup blanched finely crushed almond flour
- 1 ounce full-fat cream cheese
- 1 large egg
- 1/4 cup of heavy whipping cream
- 1/2 teaspoon of vanilla extract

Instructions

Almond flour, protein powder, half cup erythritol, baking powder, five tablespoons butter, cream cheese, and egg are all combined in a big basin. You'll get a soft, sticky dough. For 20 minutes, place the dough in the freezer. It will have sufficient firmness to roll into balls. Roll into twelve balls after wetting your hands with warm water. Into a 6-inch round baking dish, put the balls. Melt the remaining butter and erythritol in a medium pan over medium heat. Add cream and vanilla after turning the heat to low and whisk the mixture until it becomes brown. Remove from heat and whisk continuously while letting it thicken for a few minutes.

Put the baking dish into the air fryer basket while the mixture cools. The timer should be set for 6 minutes with the temperature adjusted to 320°F. Flip the monkey bread onto a platter and place it back into the baking pan when the timer dings. Sauté for 4 minutes or until the tops are fully browned. After adding the caramel sauce, let the monkey bread bake for two more minutes. Let to cool before serving.

Nutritional Values Calories: 322, Protein: 20.4g, Fat: 24.5g, Carbohydrates: 33.7g, Sugar: 0.9 g

3. Mini Cheesecake

Preparation time: 10 minutes
Cooking time: 15 minutes
Serving: 2

Ingredients

- 1 egg
- 1/2 cup of walnuts
- 2 tablespoons of salted butter
- 2 tablespoons of granular erythritol
- 4 ounces of full-fat cream cheese
- 1/2 a teaspoon of vanilla extract
- 1/8 cup of powdered erythritol

Instructions

Put butter, walnuts, and erythritol granules in a food processor. To create the dough, pulse the ingredients until they bind together. Put the dough-filled 4" springform pan into the air fryer basket. Set the thermostat to 400°F, and then set a 5-minute timer. Remove the crust and let it cool when the timer goes off. Cream cheese, egg, vanilla extract, and erythritol powder should be well combined in a medium basin. Spread the mixture over the cooked walnut crust before putting it in the air fryer basket. Set the timer for 10 minutes and raise the temperature to 300°F. After finishing, let it cool for two hours before serving.

Nutritional Values

Calories: 531, Protein: 11.4g, at: 48.3g, Carbohydrates: 31.4g, Sugar: 2.9g

4. Mini Chocolate Chip Pan Cookie

Preparation time: 10 minutes
Cooking time: 7 minutes
Serving: 4

Ingredients

- 1/2 teaspoon of unflavored gelatin
- 1/2 cup of blanched finely crushed almond flour
- 1/4 cup of powdered erythritol
- 2 tablespoons of unsalted butter (melted)
- 1 egg
- 1/2 teaspoon of baking powder
- 1/2 teaspoon of vanilla extract
- 2 tablespoons of low-carb, sugar-free chocolate chips

Instructions

Combine almond flour and erythritol in a large bowl. Gelatin, butter, and egg should all be mixed. Add vanilla and baking powder, and then stir in the chocolate chunks. Fill a 6-inch baking pan with the batter. In the air fryer basket, put the pan. The timer of the air fryer should be set for 7 minutes with the temperature adjusted to 300°F. A toothpick inserted in the middle should come out clean when the food is thoroughly cooked, and the top will be golden brown. Let it at least 10 minutes to cool.

Nutritional Values

Calories: 188, Protein: 5.6g, Fat: 15.7g, Carbohydrates: 16.8g, Sugar: 0.6 g

5. Pecan Brownies

Preparation time: 10 minutes
Cooking time: 20 minutes
Serving: 6

Ingredients

- 2 tablespoons of cocoa powder (unsweetened)
- 1/2 cup of blanched, finely ground almond flour
- 1/2 cup of powdered erythritol
- 1/2 a teaspoon of baking powder
- 1/4 cup of unsalted butter (softened)
- 1 large egg
- 1/4 cup of chopped pecans
- 1/4 cup of low-carb and sugar-free chocolate chips

Instructions

Combine almond flour, cocoa powder, erythritol and baking powder in a large basin. Add butter and egg and stir. Add chocolate chips and pecans by folding. Fill a 6-inch circular baking pan with the ingredients. In the air fryer basket, put the pan. Set the timer of the air fryer for 20 minutes and raise the temperature to 300°F.

A toothpick inserted in the middle will come out clean when the food is thoroughly cooked. Let the food 20 minutes to completely cool and set.

Nutritional Values

Calories: 215, Protein: 4.2 g, Fat: 18.9g, Carbohydrates: 21.8g, Sugar: 0.6 g

6. Blackberry Crisp

Preparation time: 5 minutes
Cooking time: 15 minutes
Serving: 4

Ingredients

- 2 cups of blackberries
- 1/3 cup of powdered erythritol
- 2 tablespoons of lemon juice
- 1/4 teaspoon of xanthan gum
- 1 cup Crunchy Granola

Instructions

Combine blackberries, lemon juice, erythritol, and xanthan gum in a big bowl. Spoon into a 6-inch-diameter round baking dish and foil it up. Could you put it in the basket of the air fryer. Set the timer for 12 minutes and raise the temperature to 350°F. Remove the foil and stir when the timer sounds. Add granola to the mixture before placing it in the air fryer basket. Set the oven to 320°F, and cook the top for 3 minutes or until golden. Serve hot.

Nutritional Values

Calories: 496, Protein: 9.2g, Fat: 42.1g, Carbohydrates: 44g, Sugar: 5.7g

7. Mug Cake

Preparation time: 5 minutes
Cooking time: 25 minutes
Serving: 1

Ingredients

- 1 egg
- 1/4 teaspoon of baking powder
- 2 tablespoons of coconut flour
- 2 tablespoons of heavy whipping cream
- 2 tablespoons of granular erythritol
- 1/4 teaspoon of vanilla extract

Instructions

Whisk the egg in a 4-inch ramekin before adding the other ingredients. Until smooth, stir. Please put it in the basket of the air fryer. Set the timer for 25 minutes and raise the temperature to 300°F. A needle should come out clean after completion. Use a spoon to eat straight out of the ramekin. Serve hot.

Nutritional Values

Calories: 237, Protein: 9.9g, Fat: 16.4g, Carbohydrates: 40.7g, sugar: 4.2g

8. Pumpkin Cookie with Frosting

Preparation time: 10 minutes
Cooking time: 7 minutes
Serving: 6

Ingredients

- 2 tablespoons of melted butter
- 1/2 cup of blanched finely crushed almond flour
- 1/2 cup of powdered erythritol (divided)
- 1 large egg

- 1/2 teaspoon of unflavored gelatin
- 1/2 teaspoon of baking powder
- 1/2 teaspoon of vanilla extract
- 1/2 teaspoon of pumpkin pie spice
- 2 tablespoons of pure pumpkin purée
- 1/2 teaspoon of ground cinnamon
- 1/4 cup low-carb, sugar-free chocolate chips
- 3 ounces of full-fat cream cheese (softened)

Instructions

Mix 1/4 cup erythritol and almond flour in a large basin. Gelatin, butter, and egg should all be mixed. Fold in chocolate chips after adding baking powder, vanilla, pumpkin pie spice, pumpkin purée, and 1/4 teaspoon cinnamon. Fill a 6-inch round baking pan with the batter. In the air fryer basket, put the pan.

The timer should be set for 7 minutes with the temperature adjusted to 300°F. A toothpick inserted in the middle should come out clean when the food is thoroughly cooked, and the top will be golden brown. Let it at least 20 minutes to cool.

Cream cheese, the last 1/4 teaspoon of cinnamon, and the final 1/4 cup of erythritol should be combined in a big bowl to produce the frosting. Beat it with an electric mixer until it puffs up. On top of the cooled biscuit, spread. If desired, add more cinnamon as a garnish.

Nutritional Values
Calories: 199, Protein: 4.8g, Fat: 16.2g, Carbohydrates: 21.5g, Sugar: 1.1g

9. Cream Cheese Danish

Preparation time: 20 minutes
Cooking time: 15 minutes
Serving: 6

Ingredients

- 3/4 cup of blanched almond flour that has been coarsely crushed
- 1 cup of mozzarella cheese, shredded
- five full-fat ounces of cream cheese, split
- 2 Egg yolks
- 3/4 cup of erythritol powder, split
- split two teaspoons of vanilla extract

Instructions

Add almond flour, mozzarella, and 1 ounce of cream cheese to a large microwave-safe bowl. After combining, microwave for one minute. Add egg yolks to the bowl after stirring. Stir consistently until soft dough develops. Add 1/2 cup erythritol and 1/4 teaspoon vanilla to the dough. To fit the basket of your air fryer, cut a piece of parchment. Using warm water on your hands, spread the dough into a rectangle that is 1/4 inch thick.

Mix the remaining cream cheese, erythritol, and vanilla in a medium bowl. Put this cream cheese mixture on the dough rectangle's right side. The dough is folded over and sealed by pressing the left side. Please put it in the basket of the air fryer. The timer should be set for 15 minutes with the temperature adjusted to 330°F. Turn the Danish over after seven minutes. Remove the Danish from the parchment when the timer goes off, and let it cool entirely before slicing.

Nutritional Values
Calories: 185, Protein: 7.4g, Fat: 14.5g, Carbohydrates: 20.8g, Sugar: 1.3g

10. Layered Peanut Butter Cheesecake Brownies

Preparation time: 20 minutes
Cooking time: 35 minutes
Serving: 6

Ingredients

- 1/2 cup of blanched finely crushed almond flour
- 1 cup powdered erythritol
- 2 tablespoons of cocoa powder (unsweetened)
- 1/2 teaspoon of baking powder
- 1/4 cup of unsalted butter (melted)
- 2 eggs (divided)
- 8 ounces full-fat cream cheese (softened)
- 1/4 cup of heavy whipping cream
- 1 teaspoon of vanilla extract
- 2 tablespoons of no-sugar-added peanut butter

Instructions

Almond flour, 1/2 cup erythritol, cocoa powder, and baking powder should all be combined in a large basin. Add butter and one egg, and stir. Into a 6-inch round baking pan, scoop the mixture. In the air fryer basket, put the pan. Set the timer for 20 minutes and raise the temperature to 300°F.

A toothpick inserted in the middle will come out clean when the food is thoroughly cooked. Let the food 20 minutes to completely cool and set. Beat the remaining 12 cups of erythritol, heavy cream, vanilla, peanut butter, and remaining egg until frothy in a large bowl. Mixture over brownies that have cooled. Reposition the pan into the air fryer basket. Set the timer for 15 minutes and raise the temperature to 300°F. Cheesecake should be mainly firm, slightly jiggling, and slightly browned when finished. After that, chill for two hours before serving.

Nutritional Values

Calories: 347, Protein: 8.3g, Fat: 30.9g, Carbohydrates: 29.8g, Sugar: 2.2g

11. Toasted Coconut Flakes

Preparation time: 5 minutes
Cooking time: 3 minutes
Serving: 4

Ingredients

- 1 cup of unsweetened coconut flakes
- 1/4 cup of granular erythritol
- 1/8 teaspoon of salt
- 2 teaspoons of coconut oil

Instructions

In a large bowl, combine oil and coconut flakes and toss to combine. Salt and erythritol should be added. Coconut flakes should be added to the air fryer basket. Set the thermostat to 300°F and start a 3-minute timer. After one minute has passed, throw the flakes. If you like more golden coconut flakes, add another minute. Keep for up to three days in an airtight container.

Nutritional Values

Calories: 165, Protein: 1.3g, Fat: 15.5g, Carbohydrates: 20.3g, Sugar: 0.5g

12. Vanilla Pound Cake

Preparation time: 10 minutes
Cooking time: 25 minutes
Serving: 6

Ingredients
- 1 cup of blanched finely crushed almond flour
- 1/4 cup of (melted) salted butter
- 2 eggs
- 1/2 cup of granular erythritol
- 1 teaspoon of vanilla extract
- 1 teaspoon of baking powder
- 1/2 cup of full-fat sour cream
- 1 ounce of full-fat cream cheese

Instructions
Combine almond flour, erythritol, and butter in a large bowl. Mix well after adding the vanilla, sour cream, baking powder and cream cheese. Add eggs, then blend. In a 6-inch round baking pan, pour the batter. In the air fryer basket, put the pan. Set the timer for 25 minutes and raise the temperature to 300°F. A toothpick in the middle of the cake will come out clean when finished. It shouldn't feel damp in the middle. The cake will crumble if you move it before it has fully cooled.

Nutritional Values
Calories: 253, Protein: 6.9g, Fat: 22.6g, Carbohydrates: 25.2g, Sugar: 1.5 g

13. Chocolate Cake

Preparation time: 10 minutes
Cooking time: 25 minutes
Serving: 6

Ingredients
- 2 eggs
- 1 cup of blanched finely crushed almond flour
- 1/4 cup of salted butter, melted
- 1/2 cup plus 1 tablespoon of granular erythritol
- 1 teaspoon of vanilla extract
- 1/4 cup of full-fat mayonnaise
- 1/4 cup of unsweetened cocoa powder

Instructions
Blend all the ingredients in a large basin. In a 6-inch round baking pan, pour the batter. Please put it in the basket of the air fryer. Set the timer for 25 minutes and raise the temperature to 300°F. A toothpick in the middle will come out clean when finished. The cake must thoroughly cool before moving; else, it will crumble.

Nutritional Values
Calories: 270, Protein: 7.0g, Fat: 25.1g, Carbohydrates: 28.8g, Sugar: 0.9g

14. Chocolate-Covered Maple Bacon

Preparation time: 5 minutes
Cooking time: 12 minutes
Serving: 2

Ingredients

- 8 slices of (sugar-free) bacon
- 1 teaspoon of coconut oil
- 1 tablespoon of granular erythritol
- 1/3 cup of low-carb, sugar-free chocolate chips
- 1/2 teaspoon of maple extract

Instructions

Put the bacon and erythritol into the air fryer basket. Set the timer for 12 minutes and raise the temperature to 350°F. Halfway through cooking, turn the bacon. Check after 9 minutes and cook till the desired doneness. (Smaller air fryers cook significantly more quickly.) Set aside the cooked bacon to cool. Coconut oil and chocolate chips should be combined in a small microwave-safe bowl. Stir after 30 seconds in the microwave. Include maple extract. Put the bacon on the parchment paper. Put the bacon in the refrigerator to chill and firm the chocolate for approximately five minutes.

Nutritional Values

Calories: 379, Protein: 15.3g, Fat: 25.9g, Carbohydrates: 31.8g, Sugar: 0.2g

15. Raspberry Danish Bites

Preparation time: 30 minutes
Cooking time: 7 minutes
Serving: 10

Ingredients

- 10 teaspoons of (sugar-free) raspberry preserves
- 1 cup of blanched finely crushed almond flour
- 1 teaspoon of baking powder
- 3 tablespoons of granular Swerve
- 2 ounces of full-fat cream cheese
- 1 large egg

Instructions

Combine all ingredients except preserves in a large basin and stir until a moist dough forms. Put the bowl in the freezer for 20 minutes to allow the dough to chill and become malleable. Ten balls of dough should be formed; gently press the center of each ball. Each ball should have 1 teaspoon of preserves in the center. To fit the basket of your air fryer, cut a piece of parchment. Put each Danish bite on the paper, flattening the bottom with a little push. Set the thermostat to 400 degrees Fahrenheit and start the timer for 7 minutes. Before transporting, let them cool fully to prevent crumbling.

Nutritional Values

Calories: 96, Protein: 3.4g, Fat: 7.7g, Carbohydrates: 9.8g, Sugar: 2.4g

16. Cinnamon Cream Puff

Preparation time: 15 minutes
Cooking time: 6 minutes
Serving: 8

Ingredients

- 1/2 teaspoon of baking powder
- 1/2 cup of blanched finely crushed almond flour
- 1/2 cup of low-carb vanilla protein powder
- 1/2 cup of granular erythritol
- 1 egg
- 5 tablespoons of unsalted butter
- 2 ounces of full-fat cream cheese
- 1/4 cup of (powdered) erythritol
- 1/4 teaspoon of ground cinnamon
- 2 tablespoons of heavy whipping cream
- 1/2 teaspoon of vanilla extract

Instructions

In a large bowl, combine almond flour, protein powder, erythritol granules, baking powder, egg, and butter; stir until a soft dough forms. For 20 minutes, place the dough in the freezer. Eight balls of dough should be formed after wetting your hands with water. To fit the basket of your air fryer, cut a piece of parchment. The dough balls should be put in batches in the air fryer basket on top of parchment paper. The timer should be set for 6 minutes with the temperature adjusted to 380°F.

Halfway through the cooking time, flip the cream puffs. Please take out the puffs and let them cool once the timer whistles. Cream cheese, erythritol powder, cinnamon, cream, and vanilla should be fluffily combined in a medium basin. Put the ingredients in a storage or pastry bag with a snipped end. Each puff should have a little opening at the bottom that you should fill with part of the cream mixture. Refrigerate for up to two days in an airtight container.

Nutritional Values Calories: 178, Protein: 14.9g, Fat: 12.1g, Carbohydrates: 22.1g, Sugar: 0.4g

17. Pan Peanut Butter Cookies

Preparation time: 5 minutes
Cooking time: 8 minutes
Serving: 8

Ingredients

- 1 egg
- 1 cup of no-sugar-added smooth peanut butter
- 1/3 cup of granular erythritol
- 1 teaspoon of vanilla extract

Instructions

Blend all the ingredients in a large basin. The liquid will start to thicken after two more minutes of stirring. Eight mixture discs should be formed by rolling them into balls and gently pressing them down. To fit your air fryer, cut a piece of parchment to size and put it in the basket. Working in batches as needed, arranging the cookies on the parchment. The timer should be set for 8 minutes with the temperature adjusted to 320°F. At the six-minute point, turn the cookies. Serve after having fully cooled.

Nutritional Values

Calories: 210, Protein: 8.8g, Fat: 17.5g, Carbohydrates: 14.1g, Sugar: 1.1g

18. Pumpkin Spice Pecans

Preparation time: 5 minutes
Cooking time: 6 minutes
Serving: 4

Ingredients

- 1/2 teaspoon of crushed cinnamon
- 1 cup of whole pecans
- 1/4 cup of granular erythritol
- 1 egg white
- 1/2 teaspoon of pumpkin pie spice
- 1/2 teaspoon of vanilla extract

Instructions

In a large bowl, mix everything until the pecans are well-coated. Please put it in the basket of the air fryer. Set the timer for 6 minutes and raise the temperature to 300°F. Cooking requires two to three tosses. Let to cool. Keep for up to three days in an airtight container.

Nutritional Values

Calories: 178, Protein: 3.2g, Fat: 17.0g, Carbohydrates: 19g, Sugar: 1.1g

19. Protein Powder Doughnut Holes

Preparation time: 25 minutes
Cooking time: 6 minutes
Serving: 12

Ingredients

- 1/2 cup of low-carb vanilla protein powder
- 1/2 cup of granular erythritol
- 1/2 teaspoon of baking powder
- 1/2 cup of blanched finely crushed almond flour
- 1 egg
- 5 tablespoons of (unsalted) butter
- 1/2 teaspoon of vanilla extract

Instructions

In a large bowl, combine each item. Put for 20 minutes in the freezer. Roll the dough into twelve balls after wetting your hands with water. To fit the basket of your air fryer, cut a piece of parchment. Doughnut holes should be put into the air fryer basket on top of parchment paper in batches as required. The timer should be set for 6 minutes with the temperature adjusted to 380°F. Halfway through cooking, turn the doughnut holes. Let to cool before serving.

Nutritional Values

Calories: 221, Protein: 19.8g, Fat: 14.3g, Carbohydrates: 23.2g, Sugar: 0.4g

30 Days Meal Plan

Intermittent fasting is something you can do when on a ketogenic diet. We'll also provide sweets to satisfy your sweet craving. You will learn about our favourite traditional low-carb dishes, including fresh salads and soups.

Average weekly calories for 150 days should be about 1500; fats between 110 and 120; carbohydrates between 20 and 40; fiber between 10 and 20; and protein between 90 and 100. We have not addded snacks but you can add snacks after counting your calories.

Day 1
Breakfast: Crustless Quiche Lorraine
Lunch: Cucumber Avocado Salad with Bacon
Dinner: Shrimp and Cauliflower

Day 2
Breakfast: Avocado & Cheese Omelet
Lunch: Keto Tots
Dinner: Stuffed Salmon

Day 3
Breakfast: Lemon & Blueberry Muffins
Lunch: Loaded Bacon-Wrapped Keto Tots
Dinner: Mustard Salmon

Day 4
Breakfast: Scotch Eggs
Lunch: Tomatoes Provençal
Dinner: Flavored Jamaican Salmon

Day 5
Breakfast: Bacon & Egg Casserole
Lunch: Crispy Brussels Sprouts
Dinner: Swordfish and Mango Salsa

Day 6
Breakfast: Eggs Scrambled with Sautéed Onions and Cheddar Cheese
Lunch: 6 oz deli ham over 2 cups mixed greens with ½ Hass avocado, 5, ½ cup of cucumbers, and 2 Tbsp blue cheese dressing
Dinner: Baked Catfish with Broccoli and Herb-Butter Blend

Day 7
Breakfast: Chorizo Breakfast Hash
Lunch: Baked Chicken Nuggets
Dinner: Salmon and Orange Marmalade

Day 8
Breakfast: Cinnamon & Egg Loaf
Lunch: Egg Salad with Lettuce
Dinner: Chili Salmon

Day 9
Breakfast: Cheese & Mushroom Egg Cups
Lunch: Stuffed Meatballs
Dinner: Salmon and Lemon Relish

Day 10
Breakfast: Raspberry & Vanilla Pancakes
Lunch: Baked Chicken Nuggets
Dinner: Halibut and Sun-Dried Tomatoes Mix

Day 11
Breakfast: Sweet "Bread" Pudding
Lunch: Crispy Brussels Sprouts
Dinner: Beet, Tomato and Goat Cheese Mix

Day 12
Breakfast: "Rice" Pudding
Lunch: Tomatoes Provençal
Dinner: Broccoli Salad

Day 13
Breakfast: Atkins Frozen Farmhouse-Style Sausage Scramble
Lunch: 1 serving Tuna-Celery Salad with Mixed Greens and 3 cherry tomatoes
Dinner: Crispy Shrimp.

Day 14
Breakfast: Scrambled Eggs with Salmon & Avocado
Lunch: Slow-Cooker Beef Chili
Dinner: Brussels sprouts and Tomatoes Mix

Day 15
Breakfast: French Toast
Lunch: Spicy Shrimp and Sausage Soup
Dinner: Brussels sprouts and Butter Sauce

Day 16
Breakfast: Bacon & Egg Muffins
Lunch: Chopped Kale Salad with Bacon Dressing
Dinner: Tasty Lamb Ribs

Day 17
Breakfast: Blueberry & Hazelnut Granola
Lunch: Sweet Potato Lunch Casserole
Dinner: Oriental Air Fried Lamb

Day 18
Breakfast: Hard-Boiled Eggs
Lunch: Air Fried Thai Salad
Dinner: Greek Beef Meatballs Salad

Day 19
Breakfast: Sausage Breakfast Sandwich
Lunch: Special Lunch Seafood Stew
Dinner: Beef Patties and Mushroom Sauce

Day 20
Breakfast: Mushroom & Spinach Frittata
Lunch: Brussels sprouts and tomatoes mix
Dinner: Lamb and Green Pesto

Day 21
Breakfast: Cauliflower Bake
Lunch: Creamy Chicken Stew
Dinner: Lamb and Spinach Mix

Day 22
Breakfast: Zucchini Fritters
Lunch: Succulent Lunch Turkey Breast
Dinner: Chili Salmon

Day 23
Breakfast: Scotch Eggs
Lunch: Stuffed Meatballs
Dinner: Beef Casserole

Day 24
Breakfast: Lemon & Blueberry Muffins
Lunch: Japanese Chicken Mix
Dinner: Lamb and Spinach Mix

Day 25
Breakfast: Spinach and Swiss Cheese Omelet
Lunch: 2 oz ham, 2 Tbsp cream cheese, and 2 dill pickle spears
Dinner: Beef Sauteed with Vegetables Over Romaine

Day 26
Breakfast: Bacon & Egg Casserole
Lunch: Bacon-Wrapped Hot Dogs
Dinner: Mustard Salmon

Day 27
Breakfast: Chorizo Breakfast Hash
Lunch: Sesame Chicken Avocado Salad
Dinner: Salmon and Lemon Relish

Day 28
Breakfast: Cinnamon & Egg Loaf
Lunch: Baked Chicken Nuggets
Dinner: Crusted Salmon

Day 29
Breakfast: Sausage Breakfast Sandwich
Lunch: Crispy Brussels Sprouts
Dinner: Stuffed Calamari

Day 30
Breakfast: French Toast
Lunch: Cucumber Avocado Salad with Bacon
Dinner: Roasted Cod and Prosciutto

Alcohol is allowed on the keto diet, but you must know how it may affect your macronutrient intake. Typically, each shot of alcohol has 100 calories (with no nutrition). Your total calorie intake will greatly affect whether you are a regular or heavy drinker. You may still follow the keto diet if you wish to avoid particular foods or have food allergies. Cutting out dairy has been demonstrated to enhance weight loss and often assists individuals in getting over a stall if they experience it while adhering to their eating plan. It's advisable to avoid snacking when using this strategy. Your meals ought to fill you up and keep you satisfied between meals. Ensure you're getting enough water to keep hydrated (and supplement with electrolytes if needed).

Review your macronutrient intake and modify your diet if you consistently feel hungry while following the recommended eating schedule. Snacking will raise your insulin level, and you want to follow the plan with as few insulin spikes as possible.

Some snacking will undoubtedly occur. You should be ready for it if they decide to get a snack. We have some fantastic keto snack ideas that you may utilize as you go.

You may substitute any meal with comparable macronutrients or add to a meal to reach the required macros for that particular meal. Even while not every dish yields a full meal, you may increase your consumption of micronutrients by using low-carb veggies. With the keto diet, vegetarianism or veganism is feasible. However, it might be challenging.

Conclusion

Let's be honest. Our greatest chance of having a healthy metabolism and an effective lifestyle is eating a nutritious diet with all the necessary nutrients. Many individuals mistakenly believe the Keto diet is just for those wanting to lose weight. You'll discover that it's just the reverse. To lower or eliminate your risk of heart disease, this diet contains heart-healthy fats like fish, olive oil, and nuts while reducing sweets and processed carbohydrates. There are strict keto diets where just 5% of the food consists of carbohydrates, 20% of the diet consists of protein and 75% of fat. Yet even a reduced version of this, which entails deliberately selecting meals rich in healthy fats and low in carbohydrates, is sufficient.

As air frying is healthier, you can cook crispy foods with very little fat using air fryers. You may adhere to a rigorous Keto diet plan and have a nice and nutritious supper. Air fryers are ideal for providing meat with a crispy appearance and superb texture in a short time.

We appreciate you reading this book. We hope it has given you enough knowledge to get started. Do not hesitate to begin. The sooner you start this diet, your health and well-being will improve. We also hope you get to try all the nutritious dishes in this book. After that, experimenting with various recipes is the next stage. Have fun on the trip!

GET YOUR BONUS

SCAN ME

Made in United States
Troutdale, OR
06/15/2023